Your Natural Diet:

Alive Raw Foods

by Dr. T. C. Fry and David Klein

Edited by David and Doris Klein

Living Nutrition Publications
Sebastopol, California

World rights reserved
Post Box 256, Sebastopol, CA 95473
Living Nutrition Online Bookstore:
www.livingnutrition.com

(707) 829-0362

Cover art by Karen Fierro
www.gardenofhealth.com
Cover design by Betsy De Gress
Printed in Canada

$15.00
ISBN 0-9717526-0-5

In loving memory of Dr. T. C. Fry
who gave many of us a healthier, happier chance at life.
1926 - 1996

For graciously contributing to
Your Natural Diet: Alive Raw Foods,
special thanks go to
Phyllis Avery, Bett Carstens, Betsy De Gress,
Katherine Dichter,
Karen Fierro, Julie Frink, Dr. Douglas Graham,
John Kohler, Paul Nison,
Jenifer Ransom, Todd Seliga, and Marti Wheeler.

Special thanks also go to Dr. Laurence Galant
for introducing me to Natural Hygiene and
the world of T. C. Fry,
Dr. Iraj Afshar for teaching me the Somatic Inquiry,
Dr. Douglas Graham for bringing this book to life,
and to my parents, Doris and Edward,
for helping me through it all.

For the love of life.

Table of Contents

Foreword

by Dr. Douglas Graham

Every once in a while a person comes along who changes the way we look at things. Dr. T. C. Fry was one of those men. T. C. has had a bigger influence on the health and eating habits of the nation than perhaps any other person. He wrote tirelessly for 25 years. Along the way, he taught many people who have themselves written best selling books, and many others who are about to. T. C. was unrelenting in his efforts to get the word out about Natural Hygiene, a lifestyle that added 25 years of robust health, that he had never experienced before, onto his life.

I count myself among the Natural Hygiene authors influenced by T. C. Included in the list are: Harvey and Marilyn Diamond, famous for their book, *Fit for Life*, Marti Wheeler, Dr. Gina Shaw, Professor Rozalind Gruben (look for her upcoming book, *Raw Nutritional Science*), and David Klein, to name just a few.

David takes his mission seriously. Having been helped to health by T. C. from a debilitating gastro-intestinal disorder (ulcerative colitis) in 1984, David Klein has become one of the world's finest health educator-writers, spreading a healthy message at every opportunity. *Your Natural Diet* is no exception. Within these pages, David has compiled his most insightful "how to" writings with much of the classic work of T. C. Fry. Taken out of context, much of this information might seem unconvincing. Taken together, *Your Natural Diet* is a powerful "how to" manual that leaves very little unsaid about creating and maintaining vibrant health through healthful eating and living practices.

If you are ready to become truly influenced by natural health sense, *Your Natural Diet* is for you. If you are interested in achieving top level health, cutting straight to the chase and replacing your old self-destructive habits with self-constructive ones, read this deeply illuminating book. If you want to chew on food for thought that will challenge your beliefs and encourage you to improve yourself, David Klein has put together a winner for you.

Your Natural Diet is must reading for any true health enthusiast. In a time of dime a dozen health fads where new diet programs and gimmicks are being promoted every day, *Your Natural Diet* offers timeless teaching brought to you by two of the world's masters. *Your Natural Diet* is a book for the ages. Read it and enjoy, read it and grow healthier.

Dr. Douglas Graham is President of Healthful Living International and author of Grain Damage, On Nutrition and Physical Performance, The High Energy Diet Recipe Guide, Perpetual Health, and Hygienic Fasting.
www.doctorgraham.com

Introduction

by David Klein

One magical evening in 1984 my mind exploded. I was studying the *Natural Hygiene Course*, which was masterminded by Dr. T. C. Fry, and understood how to save and resurrect my life. I also understood what humanity needed to undo disease, suffering and its descent toward extinction. My revelation of health via the principles of natural raw food diet and self healing set in motion my rapid healing and lit a fire in me which is still raging on. From an abyss on the brink of destruction to the pinnacle of health, here I am!

Some people describe my passion for getting people the messages of raw food eating and self healing as driven and indomitable. A minute has rarely gone by in twenty years when I have not been caught up in thinking of ways to effectively present this information so that everyone can understand and embrace it. Where is this passion coming from? From my desire to help others after recovering from eight years of my own hellacious suffering, my will to live in a healthy body and enjoy the fruits of life, and to see my fellow Earth beings realize the same. No one deserves to suffer!

Anyone who knows me knows that I'll be educating the world for the next hundred years, or as long as it takes for humanity to wake up to healthful living. I love doing this work—empowering people with this knowledge and seeing them overcome suffering, thwarting death, and becoming healthy and liberated from the medical traps is heartening and exhilarating! Every woman, man and child deserves to live a healthful life in a healthy body! The information describing how to heal, rejuvenate and regenerate is here and available to everyone now and it is high time that everyone gets it! As Thomas Henry Huxley said, "Education is the instruction of the intellect in the laws of Nature." Natural *is* the way to be!

Humanity needs to know that:

- We are biological (not technological or medical) creatures; natural is the way.
- Our biological/physiological dietetic constitution is frugivore.
- Alive raw fruits, succulent plants, seeds and nuts are the foods which constitute our natural, most delicious and most healthful diet; "live foods for live people" is the watchword.
- Cooking food is an act of destruction, creating toxins; cooked meat and grains are carcinogenic.
- Every nutrient we need is available in fruit and plant foods; there is no need to kill and eat dead animals.
- A meal of three apples is immeasurably nutritionally superior to any cooked food meal. Simple eating is not boring—it is deliciously liberating and reverses aging!
- Our bodies know how to self heal disease—we merely have to step out of the way, live on simple raw juices, and/or fruits and vegetables, or on water, get rest and sleep and the body will detoxify and heal.
- Germs do not cause illness—they are all beneficial, working symbiotically with the body to help digest plant foods, synthesize some vitamins and clean up wastes.
- We cannot become healthy if we attempt to drug and continue to pollute our bodies with medicines and dead deranged "foods."
- Every drug or medicine is poison and has no healing power.
- There are no quick fixes or short cuts to health—only the body itself can regenerate a healthier body, and it needs a clean diet and supportive conditions to accomplish that.
- Relying on outside modalities for healing disempowers us; relying on Providence for self healing is the way to actualize perfect health and maximum longevity.
- There are no mysteries behind why we get sick—the information describing the cause of and way to overcome every illness, and the proper professional help, is here and available to everyone.
- Disease is not inevitable or out of our control—we only become diseased if we poison and enervate ourselves.

• No one need fear "getting sick." "Sickness" is nature's way of detoxifying and telling us that we need to correct our thinking and live more healthfully.

• Perfect health and joyous living are our birthright, and we can all move toward their realization every day, on the glorious healthful living path.

I thank you for reading this and for anything you can do to spread the message of healthful living. I am eternally grateful for my mentor, Dr. T. C. Fry, who provided the opportunity to share this information with you.

There is a universal spiritual law which says that to receive we must give. It follows that for every ounce of good will we put out toward our fellow Earth citizens, we will receive more enrichment in return. This is so true! It feels so good to give—to oneself by creating a healthier body, and to humanity by sharing this information. This raises our and Mother Earth's level of health and deepens our spiritual connection, becoming a joyous daily ritual or celebration. The fruits of this healing work are simply *the fruits of life*. I love sharing with you and wish you joyful health and endless abundance.

* * *

Notice to Reader

The following manuscript contains writings by Dr. T. C. Fry and David Klein, with contributions by others taken from *Living Nutrition Magazine*. Writings where the author is not noted are by T. C. Fry. Dr. Fry's works are re-printed by Living Nutrition Publications with his permission.

1

Some of the Enormous Benefits You Can Expect From Your Natural Diet and Healthful Practices

Based soundly and scientifically upon our natural biological disposition—upon our natural physical, mental, emotional, sensory and spiritual needs—you can expect sensational improvements when you eat a raw diet and practice the totally effective health system of which it is a part. The health system of which the natural raw food diet is a part is the basis for vibrant, sickness-free well-being! By following this natural and effective system in practice, you almost surely will:

1. Overcome, once and for all time, occasional illnesses or annoying ailments. Whether it be indigestion, colds, flu bouts, mucus expectoration, headaches, backaches, fevers and "itises" or even such "incurable" problems as acne, allergy, arthritis, asthma, constipation, heart and cardiovascular problems, herpes, psoriasis, skin problems, sinusitis, tinnitus, tumors or whatever, this systems enables you to overcome almost anything simply by discontinuing and removing easily recognized causes, and establishing conditions that build great health.

2. Because you'll discontinue and avoid easily recognizable causes of discomforts, sicknesses and disease, you need not suffer even so much as another case of indigestion, aches and pains, fever (itis), sore throat, cough, cold or anything else!

3. Normalize your weight if it is excessive. Without dieting or counting calories, the Natural Hygiene or Healthful Living regimen born of properly meeting our needs causes the overweight to

quickly, naturally, safely, surely, and permanently lose down to a naturally normal weight set-point.

4. Eliminate physicians, hospitals, drugs, and nostrums from your and your family's lives. You'll also be spared their astronomical costs as well as the aches, pains, discomforts, agonies, and lost time.

5. Save thousands of dollars every year in food, energy, medical, hospital, drug, labor, insurance, and other outlays!

6. Energize yourself! You'll get more done when your energy levels go up! You become more lovable and charming as you become happier, more radiant and more dynamic.

7. Increase your brainpower and mental alertness. Your thinking will be clearer, sharper and more focused. Your IQ and wisdom will increase significantly.

8. Have new-found strength, stamina, vigor and vitality.

9. Enjoy clearer complexion with a glowing and radiant skin tone.

10. Speak with an improved voice that tends to bell clearness.

11. Restore yourself to relative youth! You'll look, act and feel up to 20 years younger within one to four months.

12. Eliminate most digestive problems within 24 hours after going on this marvelous diet.

13. Improve your productivity and job performance, thus increasing your income appreciably.

14. Feel like a million! You'll have a buoyancy and bounce that even younger people do not have!

15. Decrease your sleep needs by about an hour daily even though you'll be better slept, more alert, and better rested.

16. You'll be sharper, more precise and correct in your judgments and assessments, thus enabling you to more accurately and quickly perform both physical and mental tasks.

17. When you start doing what you should always have been doing, you'll start being what you always should have been! When you do right, you'll become right.

The enormity of the task of persuasion

I have written this in the hope that you will apply it so as to become a happy, caring, charming, lovable, loving, highly competent and brainier human being. I know I have quite a task in view of the many erroneous concepts which most of us subscribe to—concepts that may subconsciously close your mind to many truths.

The most difficult of tasks is to present the truth to those programmed in misconceptions and errors so as to win its acceptance. Especially is this so when seemingly impossible benefits are promised.

I feel my efforts here to be along that line—how to present to you the truths about diet, health and well-being so as not to offend your sensibilities at their present level nor risk your dismissal as ridiculous in comparison with currently accepted and perpetuated errors—errors that have made America one of the most disease-ridden nations on earth—a country of 260 million people who spend more on "disease care" than the next two billion highest spenders altogether! Despite this, our over one trillion dollar annual "health care" bill continues to escalate and compound at about 16% per year, self-evidence that our health is getting worse for all that.

Appropriately, it has been observed that truth is often stranger than fiction. Indeed, it is! For, herein, you'll find that what is true seems too good to be true. Remember, only that which is true can yield good!

While I have largely mastered the art of presenting truths in terms that are self-evident—simply undeniable by rational and thinking individuals—I find many who have been so steeped in errors and misconceptions that they reject truths that are plainly obvious.

Prevention impossible and unnecessary

Thus, in telling you that our natural diet prevents diseases, I am, in effect, saying that an unnatural diet causes disease. This happens to be the truth. No amount of "prevention" works if causes are there!

I feel a bit of clarification is in order in the use of the prevention. It is not necessary to prevent that which will not happen unless caused! So, in reality, the natural diet prevents nothing—the term prevent is used in the present day context. Disease is regarded as inevitable but can be prevented with vaccinations, certain foods with certain vitamins, minerals, antioxidants, and so on. These agencies prevent nothing (except deficiency) if causes still prevail. Discontinuing and removing causes prevents everything.

An auto performs well on the gasoline for which its engine is designed. It will perform poorly on kerosene and will all the sooner clog up and conk out, even ruining the engine. In the same light, the human body thrives on the dietary regimen to which it is naturally adapted while it will perform poorly on an unnatural diet—yes, even conk out. On an unnatural diet the body will suffer illnesses, impairments and impediments that lead to early incapacitation and death.

In this book you'll learn that humans became adapted to a particular diet just as did other creatures of nature. You do not have to believe this. Your own inherent instincts are still alive and well and will unerringly determine this natural diet if you ask yourself certain questions.

You'll learn that most conventionally eaten foods not only fail to furnish needed nutrients but actually intoxicate the body directly and indirectly via intestinal flora. This leads to both deficiencies and sicknesses. The body is weakened and impaired from deficiency while it is forced into emergency cleansing crises called illnesses when saturated with toxicants and morbid matters. Continuation of unhealthy practices leads to chronic problems and irreversible impairments.

Junky foods make junky bodies!

You'll learn that cooked foods are a curse in the human body. They are contrary to our natural endowments—nature did not equip us with cook stoves. Cooked foods epitomize our love affair with disease-causing, and life-sapping fare.

You'll learn that heated oils, fats, proteins, starches and sugars are all carcinogenic.

You'll learn that overeating is caused by stresses, distresses, and by a body driven in a mad quest for nutrients that are deficient or missing in the diet eaten.

You'll learn that unnatural and deficient foods distress the body, hence invokes the "feast against famine" response, thus causing gross overeating and unnatural weight gain.

You'll learn about foods that have high biological value and those that are negative in their health values.

You'll learn about negative calorie foods—the more you eat, the more of your fat reserves the body uses to supply the energy necessary to process them and operate your body. Most of these foods are quite nutritious otherwise.

I wrote this to inspire and motivate you to do what is necessary to realize wonderful health and radiant well-being. I want you and every human being to be a superb example of:

1. Vibrant sickness-free health.
2. A lovely, loving, caring, and charming person.
3. An attractively fit individual.
4. A person bubbling over with energy.
5. A person of keen mind and intellect.
6. The personification of goodness and happiness.
7. In short, a person who realizes the bountiful potential with which you are naturally endowed.

I have striven to present you with the touchstones necessary to become this noble being.

2
What is Diet?

A diet consists of all the foodstuffs eaten. In reality, everything that the body uses from the outside for nutritive processes should be included as part of the diet. This means that water, oxygen and sunshine, though not regarded as foodstuffs, are also part of the diet!

Foods are the raw materials of life. There are other vital needs for life. However, most of us flunk in the game of life by failing to properly furnish the body with its nutrient needs.

Up front, I want you to know that this book is about natural (Godmade) foods.

What do our dietary authorities teach?

The medical system teaches that, by and large, diet is an unimportant consideration as a causative or restorative factor in disease. They do not, by and large, bother with dietary guidance or even suggest that dietary indiscretions are the primary cause of our suffering. They have been miseducated by drug supported medical institutions to look for hobgoblins—germs, viruses, and now bad genes—to be fought with deadly drugs or expensive therapies!

Medical practitioners are exalted in our cartel controlled press, TV, and other communications media as authorities upon about everything when, in fact, they are the biggest dupes and dopes around! (The use of the word dopes is deliberate—drug addiction among medical professionals is 44 times greater than among the general populace!).

Medical personnel are praised by the media as heroes and heroines because TV, newspapers and other media are owned and controlled by those who own and control the medical/drug complex. They seek fealty and patronage from those who they maneuver and manipulate into sickness, disease and general mediocrity.

Miseducated medical practitioners are not merely failures—the burgeoning disease bills and the growing army of diseased and suffering attest to that—but actually cause many of the problems for which dietary practices are not responsible.

Dietitians as providers of customers to the medical industry!

The dietary and nutritional professions teach the Basic Five Food Groups as the basis for nutrient adequacy. Indeed, nutrient adequacy is all that we need from a diet—even if a single food furnishes it all! And many of our natural foods are nutritionally adequate within themselves! Like a Californian who lived in excellent health on grapes alone! Like a Floridian who lived in excellent health for six years on oranges alone! Like thousands here and there in the tropics who thrive on one to a few fruits all their lives.

Even more important than nutrient adequacy is this first commandment of eating: "Thou shalt not poison thyself."

The Basic Five food groups grossly violates the first commandment in four of the five food groups it teaches us to consume! So atrocious and pathogenic (disease-causing) is the conventional dietetic and nutritional fare advocated by the professionals that it is, within context, responsible for more than 95% of our country's ills!

The basic five food groups consist of the following

1. MILK AND DAIRY PRODUCTS. All such products are totally unfit for human consumption! All are outside the natural human diet. All are pathogenic! They would never be consumed in a state of nature. Only human milk is for humans!

2. The so-called PROTEIN group includes all meats and that means poultry and fish, eggs, legumes (beans, peas and peanuts), nuts and seeds. Nuts and seeds can be eaten raw and are of benefit in the human diet if their acid end-products are offset with vegetables. Some fresh peas and beans can be eaten raw with benefit, too. In nature we would consume very little nuts and seeds. All the

rest of this category are abominations in the human diet and would never be consumed in a state of nature.

3. The GRAIN group with its many products like breads, pastries, pastas, etc. Grains included in this group are wheat, rice, corn (maize), oats, rye, barley and millet. Needless to say, the entire grain group, except for sweet corn, which is technically a fruit, is unfit for human consumption and would never be consumed in a state of nature. Likewise, it is disease-causing no matter how eaten.

4. Lumped together as a group are FRUITS AND VEGETABLES when both have a widely divergent dietary character.

Commonly called vegetables are fruits like tomatoes, eggplants, cucumbers, squash and peppers. Anything that ripens when its seeds are viable are fruits! Fruits are that part of a seed package created by tree, stalk or vine to attract consumption by a biological symbiont for the purpose of distributing its seeds, thus insuring procreation of kind.

Also called vegetables are tubers, roots and bulbs like potatoes, yams, carrots, beets, turnips, taro, kohlrabi, radishes, onions, leeks and so on.

Further, cultivated grasses and weeds like lettuce, cabbage family members, kale, collards, spinach, chards, broccoli, cauliflower, and greens generally are called vegetables. Certain of these foods are beneficial in the diet and some have toxic substances!

What is generally referred to as fruits are bananas, apples, oranges and citrus family members, grapes, berries, cherries, mangos, peaches, apricots, papayas, pineapples and much more.

Fruits that are rarely mentioned as fruits are melons—that is, cantaloupes, honeydews, muskmelons and watermelons. Pumpkins and any seed-bearing package which ripens usually have a food complement to attract consumption with the incidental benefit of the discarding of the seeds away from the parent plants. Fruits are among our best foods. With uncanny intelligence, they were created by plant life to meet the exact nutrient needs of their biological symbionts—nectar for bees would be a good example.

In nature you would consume most fruits with gusto. These

are, of course, our natural foods. There are isolated groups of people today who live entirely on fruits and some who live almost totally on a single fruit staple, notably some banana and plantain eating peoples.

5. The fifth food group receives little or no mention from nutritionists, though they and dietitians included many of this group's items daily in their recipes and meals. Some call the fifth food group Accessory Foods. These include salt, sugar, pepper, condiments, candies, syrups, wines, beers, jellies, jams, vinegar and a raft of other pernicious products. Again, no so-called foods in this category should ever be touched by human lips!

Why should nutritionists and dietitians recommend and urge that we consume servings from each food category on a daily basis? The truth is that, like physicians, they are mere dupes and largely miseducated puppets in the matter. What most have been taught is not only unscientific and invalid, but responsible for the mostly diseased and ailing American populace. Our commercial masters who endow our educational institutions and pay for most advertising control the American dietary profession and almost totally determine the pathogenic American diet.

Even more incredible is the fact that our secret super rich masters want us all to be mediocre, unthinking and unquestioning. Like the Roman slaves, we are to be totally diverted with "bread and circuses."

These so-called food groups have nothing to do with proper nutrition! It is obvious to the knowledgeable and observant that they are mere commercial divisions of the marketplace! The super rich own and control food industries. They also control government and educational institutions. They have devious, diabolical and monstrous goals for the bulk of the populace.

In view of our induced national infatuation with the fare of these so-called food groups, most of which are pathogenic, the use of the word incredible when referring to our beneficent natural diet is understandable and justified.

Most of us have never heard of the natural foods of humans

mentioned or referred to as such. Lies, errors, misrepresentations and calumnies are spewed forth as science to our peoples about our natural dietary (of mostly fruits), while pathogenic fare is praised as if it were manna from heaven!

In view of our statements that the diet we pinpoint *through your instincts* as natural to humans prevents all diseases and are key to overcoming all remediable diseases—in view of the insidious beliefs cultivated about diet and nutrition in America—it is very appropriate that we use the word incredible when describing our natural diet.

3
What is Nutrition?

The science of nutrition embraces all that contributes to the nurture of organisms. Nutrition is concerned with that which nourishes the human body. As well, this science concerns itself with the many bodily activities and processes whereby needed nutrients are appropriated, digested, absorbed, assimilated, and utilized.

About 90% of our bodies' nutrient needs, aside from water, are for caloric foods that the body uses for energy and heat needs. If not used as fats, all caloric values are used as sugars: fructose and glucose. Mitochondria or organelles (there are a few hundred in blood cells and up to 50,000 of these life units within well-developed muscle cells) convert these sugars with oxygen into adenosine triphosphate (ATP). The body uses ATP much like a gun uses gunpowder—instant energy upon command or demand.

The body also breaks down its fats and uses them for its energy and heat needs. Fats are used for these purposes only when sugars are not available.

About 4% to 5% of our bodies' nutrient needs, aside from water, are for amino acids. Note that I said amino acids, not proteins! Proteins from outside the body are alien substances that distress it if injected directly into the bloodstream. Many proteins, like egg whites, can cause anaphylactic shock and instant death if injected into the vital system. If we eat proteins, the body must laboriously digest them and absorb the resulting amino acids. In our natural foods, proteins come to us predigested as amino acids!

Our bodies can use ONLY amino acids or digest and use proteins that have not been heated—amino acids start to be destroyed at 118 degrees Fahrenheit and virtually all are destroyed at 160 degrees, the temperature of pasteurization. At this temperature, almost all proteins are disorganized and deranged with most amino acids already deaminated.

About 3% of our bodies' nutrient needs, aside from water, are for mineral matter, that is, organized or organic mineral matter as it occurs within the context of raw foods. Inorganic minerals as in supplements, food additives, metals, ores, rocks, soil, sea water and cooked foods are poisonous! For example, iodine is a vital nutrient. The body must get it from plant sources. Inorganic iodine bears the skull and cross-bones in a pharmacy. All inorganic minerals are toxic! This applies to all inorganic minerals such as sodium, iron (causes hemochromatosis and hepatitis), magnesium, chlorine, phosphorus, potassium, calcium (results in kidney stones, plaques, clogging materials, etc.) and about 40 other minerals which, in organic context, the body must have to meet its nutrient needs.

Heating foods expands the cells and their contents, causing minerals to be deranged from their natural context and spilled into the liquid medium as inorganic ashes. Cooking renders minerals unavailable for body use—they become toxic debris instead. The fact that they are a primary cause of leukocytosis in their organic form in hard water and sea water attest to this.

About 1% to 2% of the body's needs, aside from water in foods, are for essential fatty acids. At one time these were named as linoleic (popularly called omega-6), linolenic (popularly referred to as omega-3), and arachidonic. Now it has been found that only linoleic is an essential fatty acid because the body can synthesize all other fatty acids needed. The reason something is called essential is because the body cannot synthesize it. The reason the body does not have the ability to synthesize it is because it is so reliably plentiful in natural foods there is no need for the capability.

A small fraction of 1% of the body's needs are for a fifth category of nutrients called vitamins. The need is so small that, if you took all your vitamin needs for a whole year and added them together, they would not fill a sewer's thimble! However, they are absolutely vital in human nutrition for all that.

Heat deranges and destroys vitamins at rather low temperatures. As most cooking is at high temperatures, above the boiling point, most cooked foods are not only virtually worthless but give us a double whammy with their toxic debris.

There are miscellaneous nutrients the body may use called auxones and hormones. However, little is in the literature about these compounds.

The study of nutrition revolves largely around these nutrients. Physiology and other health sciences treat other aspects of nutrition. Nutritionists usually spend four to eight years learning their profession. For all that, we'd be much better off without them. Proper nutrition should concern itself only with consuming foods to which we are naturally adapted.

"It is better to be ignorant than to have learned so much that isn't so!"

The science of correct feeding

Most of us don't want to know about science. Somehow we have the impression that it is complex and sophisticated in the areas it is applied. But science is really very simple!

Science is observation and ascertainment of the principles and facts in a given area. Science means applying these to maximal advantage. Obviously, that which works is scientific. Just as plainly, that which does not work is unscientific.

When our unnatural diet is responsible for diseases and suffering, evidently the unnatural diet is unscientific, that is, not in accord with science because it fails to meet the requirements of humans. Additionally, an unnatural diet intoxicates its eaters. This give rise to sicknesses, ailments and diseases.

Does our present system of feeding work? If we attribute our present pathology even in part to dietary practices, then our present system of feeding is errant. Nature (God) never imposed suffering upon animals or humans as a condition of existence. The Bible calls for only fruits as our diet per Genesis, 1:29:30.

Our subject, correct feeding, is called orthophagy or correct nutrition (orthotrophy) if you want to use rather obscure language as "scientists" are apt to do.

4

How Our Natural Diet
Leads to Wellness

Because a raw diet of mostly fruits with daily vegetable salads, some nuts and seeds and very small amounts (less than a teaspoon daily) of sea vegetation is replete with all our nutrient needs, we suffer no deficiencies.

Because this raw food dietary is "clean-burning," that is, has little or no toxic substances within themselves or as by-products after ingestion—that is, no disease-causing factors—discomforts and suffering will not be a result.

The body's vital energies, if enough rest and sleep are obtained, will be sufficient to cope with some of the toxic factors in vegetables. For instance, lettuces have lactucarium, a milky soporific and mild opiate. Cabbage family members have sulfur compounds that are mildly toxic. For a rather complete listing of toxic substances (carcinogens) in foods, I suggest that you go to the library and look up the September 23, 1983 issue of *Science* magazine.

I also suggest that you refer to the book, *Diet, Nutrition and Cancer* published in 1982 by the Nutritional Research Council. Chapter 13 of this book lists so many pathogenic effects of cooked foods you'll swear off cooked foods forever out of respect for the temple of your being, your magnificent body.

Yes, a raw diet enables you to overcome diseases!

If you adopt a natural diet of raw foods, your body can easily cope with cleansing itself of past toxic accumulations and normalize its weight. While there may be some discomforts because of heavy detoxification occasioned by an improved diet and regimen, especially from emptying the fat cells which are often "under the rug" storage depots for toxins and morbid matters, the overall improvements will be nothing less than spectacular down line.

Sicknesses, diseases and ailments will cease because their underlying causes have been discontinued, removed and eliminated. The body is totally self-healing and will do so if not burdened with new toxic input. Only irreversible organic damage cannot be overcome—problems like Alzheimer's, where significant brain cell loss has been sustained.

* * *

Detoxification

by David Klein

Many, if not most people, begin transitioning to a raw food diet when they are severely ill; some do so when they are attempting to recover from minor nagging illness symptoms; and still others make the change when they are free of symptoms. In all of these conditions, once the body begins to assimilate a higher proportion of natural raw foods, it initiates detoxification and health-building actions since it is always striving to establish a higher state of wellness.

The new, enzymatically-active live raw foods with their nutritious, energizing sugars cause the body to spring into action, utilizing much of its energy in cleaning house and repairing itself: purging debris, shedding old inferior cells, and using the new raw nutrients to build a completely new, healthier body. It is recommended that the transition be made gradually, to avoid triggering the uncomfortable symptoms that can accompany a drastic cleansing process. As long as there is vitality, the opportunity exists for the body to rejuvenate to a far more vigorous level of health. Results are often noticed within 24 hours of beginning a new healthful regimen.

Detoxification is a self-purifying process which the body carries out at all times, but most aggressively during the early to late morning hours. It is advantageous to eat lightly in the morning. Heavy foods eaten at this time suspend the cleansing process, keeping us toxic, and, in some cases, overweight. The process of "detox" entails: 1. the cells off-loading metabolic wastes and environmental toxins into the bloodstream for filtering by the liver and kidneys for elimination, and 2. the organs of elimination (bowels, kidneys, lungs, skin, vagina) releasing metabolic, environmental and residual food wastes via feces, urine, breath, sweat and menses. Toxins are also expectorated in mucus via the throat and sinuses.

Under normal conditions of healthful living and natural diet, the body is able to eliminate metabolic wastes and other environmental pollutants through its normal organs of elimination. However, under chronic excessive bombardment with unnatural dietary fare, environmental pollutants, emotional stress, and/or overeating on even good natural foods, the body's eliminative capacities are not equal to the task, and a buildup of toxins increases as the days and years go by. This condition, called toxicosis, leads to accelerated aging, fatigue, illness, and, in many cases, to obesity. In this condition of toxicity, which is particularly likely if one has lived on a diet of foods such as cooked meat, dairy, bread, and junk foods, the body harbors sticky and insoluble debris and waste matter on artery and bowel walls, as well as in the bloodstream, tissues, bowels, and organs.

Fortunately, the body is a magnificently designed masterpiece of self-regulation and self-healing, always striving to establish and maintain purity and wellness. When a toxic load becomes too dangerous for the body, it intelligently enacts a detoxification/elimination/purging/housecleaning event or phase, manifested by any of these "symptoms": sore throat, inflammation, fever, skin outbreaks, coated tongue, mucus expectoration, body aches, nausea, vomiting, and diarrhea. Malodorous body wastes and underarms are signs that toxic, putrid, fermented matter and acids are being eliminated. During the detoxification phase, many people experience lightheadedness and headaches as the body stirs up and dumps toxins into the bloodstream for processing and elimination. During a thorough detox, unhealthy fat, cysts and even tumors are also broken down (autolyzed) and eliminated. As toxins are stirred up and released, the body relaxes and people also typically experience short-term symptoms of mental-emotional detox: mood swings, depression, sadness, anger, and crying.

When the organs of elimination are weak and/or overloaded, the body will resort to eliminating toxins through any convenient outlet it can find: e.g., the eyes, ears, throat, vagina, skin (sweating, rashes and suppurations), sinuses, and scalp. When we experience any of these signs of elimination, we typically feel fatigued and sleepy, as the body is directing much of its energy toward accomplishing the housecleaning. At such times, it is always wise to assist the body by heeding the calls for extra rest and sleep. All of these "symptoms" will diminish and then vanish when the body is sufficiently cleaned out, providing we adhere to a healthful lifestyle regimen.

In conjunction with the heightened detoxification action, the body works at repairing any damage, regenerating new cells, rejuvenating and restoring wellness. The repair work mostly occurs when we sleep. When there is damage to be repaired and rejuvenation to be accomplished, the body needs extra sleep. We typically feel weak and need plenty of extra sleep in the beginning stage of the rejuvenation phase. If the toxemia, physical damage, degeneration and emotional distress is severe, this phase may last for weeks or months. It is important to understand that the symptoms of the detoxification and rejuvenation process signify the workings of the awesome rejuvenative power of the body. It will help the process if we appreciate the workings of the body and do everything possible to assist it in its healing processes. We can do this by taking a break or a sabbatical from our normal routines, obtaining plenty of extra sleep and rest—if necessary, complete rest—as well as eating simply, until the work is sufficiently accomplished and we experience new vigor and vitality. In many cases it would be ideal to take the sabbatical at a comfortable health center or retreat with fasting supervision, juicing, deep rest and hygiene education.

If we persevere through the uncomfortable detox symptoms, get extra sleep and rest when feeling tired or unwell, and resist covering up symptoms with medicines (which only add more toxins to the system), we will arrive at a wonderful state of well being in the quickest time possible, and in the process, we will learn invaluable lessons about how the body works to restore health. Some of the rewards include freedom from illness, sweet smelling breath, no body odors, easy and inoffensive elimination, shinier, thicker hair, clearer eyes and skin, more mental energy and clarity, better memory, more joie de vivre, slimmer belly, no cellulite, greater stamina, deeper connection to spirit, and finding a mutual attraction with healthy, vivacious people like ourselves. Through healthful living practices which keep our bodies clean inside and free of energy-robbing toxic matter, we can ensure a healthier, longer, more vital and youthful life, free ourselves from disease and aging, and tap into the wellspring of joy within.

* * *

Your Gift

by David Klein

You have a magnificent self-healing body -
you have it all.
Your body knows how to heal itself -
it is trying to do so now.
Give your body the proper care it needs -
allow your body to completely heal itself, and it will.

5

How An Unnatural Diet Causes Diseases

Just as kerosene fouls up an automobile or airplane engine which was not designed for it, so too will foods foul up human bodies if they are not adapted to them. If you are not physiologically adapted to a diet, it will be repulsive to you in its raw natural state—you cannot relish the food nor sustain yourself on it in good health. When you eat an unnatural diet by artifice, that is, by denaturing it by cooking and modifying and camouflaging its taste with condiments and so on, you are doing the following:

1. Heat deranging and destroying the nutrients within the food.

2. Deranging your taste buds through excitation with toxic substances to make the unpalatable food acceptable. All poisonous substances impose burdensome eliminative problems upon the body. Sicknesses, ailments and diseases result.

3. Causing nutrient deficiencies by eating a partially or wholly nutrient deranged "food."

4. Causing protein malnutrition. Cooking destroys proteins and amino acids. Once oxidized and destroyed by cooking, you can no longer derive any benefit from proteinaceous substances other than, perhaps "empty calories," that is, nutrient-bereft fuel. Once oxidized, proteins are soil (food) for bacteria which putrefy (rot) it. Bacterial putrefactive by-products are highly toxic and carcinogenic. These by-products are methane gas (the source for smelly gas emissions when you eat beans, for instance), hydrogen sulfide and mercaptans (which yield the rotten egg smell when carried out by the methane gas), cadaverine, putrescine, ammonias, indoles, skatoles, leukomaines and profusion of other toxic and carcinogenic substances.

5. Laying the groundwork for putrefactive bacterial flora that will vitiate your intestinal tract. Eaters of cooked foods and wrong foods have about two pounds of bacterial flora up and down their digestive tracts. Raw food eaters have only a few ounces.

6. Laying the groundwork for alcohol and vinegar poisoning. Heated sugars and carbohydrates are readily fermented by fungi and bacteria with, first, alcohol as a by-product and then vinegar which is dozens of times more toxic than alcohol.

7. Intoxicating your body with the toxic debris (deranged nutrients) of what once had nutrient value. Instead of materials your body can use, you have toxins that put the body into a frenzy and, if overwhelmed by the toxic load, into a pathological state.

As you can see, cooked foods and condiments (most condiments are toxic plant excitants and stimulants: life-sapping inorganic substances like salt, pathogenic fermentation products like soy sauces, cheeses, etc.) are a curse to our well-being.

There are many toxic substances that are commonly eaten. For instance:

1. Ordinary commercial orange juice contains a carcinogen! Because the whole orange is squeezed, the toxic limonene (a volatile and flammable oil) in the skin is in the juice. The same goes for lemon and grapefruit juices. Refer to the Office of Toxicological Sciences of the Food and Drug Administration (FDA).

2. Ordinary mushrooms contain several toxic substances (mainly hydrazine) that are carcinogenic. Refer to the September 23, 1983 issue of *Science* magazine.

3. Tofu, a highly refined soy bean product, contains several carcinogens, notably indole and nitropyrene. Refer to *Diet, Nutrition and Cancer.*

4. Alfalfa sprouts contain a carcinogen, canavanine. Refer to the September 23, 1983 issue of *Science,* and the FDA's Office of Toxicological Sciences.

5. All cooked and heated oils and fats as in fried foods, nuts, seeds, meats, etc. contain deadly carcinogens. Their aerated fumes are worse in the lungs than tobacco smoke! Refer to *Diet, Nutri-*

tion and Cancer.

The list seems endless! We Americans poison ourselves so much that we have more health problems per capita than any other country on earth. More than 16% of our national wealth goes down the disease rat hole.

Needless to say, all discomforts, illnesses and suffering are abnormal, unnatural and unnecessary.

Is cooked food good for us?

In nature all animals eat living foods as yielded up by nature. Only humans cook their foods and only humans suffer widespread sicknesses and ailments. Those humans who eat mostly living foods are more alert, think clearer, sharper and more logically and become more active. Best of all, live food eaters become virtually sickness-free!

Cooking is a process of food destruction from the moment heat is applied to the foodstuff. Long before dry ashes results, food values are totally destroyed. If you put your hand just for a moment into boiling water or on a hot stove, that should forever persuade you just how destructive heat is. Food is usually subjected to these destructive temperatures for perhaps half an hour or more. What was living substance becomes totally dead very rapidly with exposure to heat!

Cooking renders food toxic! The toxicity of the deranged debris of cooking is confirmed by the doubling and tripling of white blood cells after eating a cooked food meal. The white blood cells are the first line of defense and are, collectively, popularly called "the immune system."

As confirmed by hundreds of researches cited in the prestigious National Academy of Science's National Research Council's book, *Diet, Nutrition and Cancer,* all cooking quickly generates mutagens and carcinogens in foods.

Proteins begin coagulating and deaminating at temperatures commonly applied in cooking, and are devoid of nutritive value.

Vitamins are rather quickly destroyed by cooking.

Minerals quickly lose their organic context and are returned to their native state as they occur in soil, sea water and rocks, metals and so on. In such a state they are unusable and the body often shunts them aside where they may combine with saturated fats and cholesterol in the circulatory system, thus clogging it up with cement-like plaque.

Heated fats are especially damaging because they are altered to form acroleins, free radicals and other mutagens and carcinogens as confirmed in *Diet, Nutrition and Cancer.*

Thus you can see that dead foods make dull, diseased and sooner dead people.

How osteoporosis is caused

As an example of the modus operandi of disease causation, let's look at a widespread problem called osteoporosis, that is, bone porosity where bones lose their structural strength and present a Swiss cheese like appearance under the microscope. How do bones lose calcium and other minerals so that this condition results?

Bones are composed of mostly alkaline minerals, calcium being the primary mineral. The body maintains a homeostatic condition whereby blood, tissues and fluids are virtually all of an alkaline pH of 7.40. If the pH varies significantly from this operating alkaline homeostasis, it goes into a coma and death may ensue. Both alkalosis and acidosis can be deadly.

The body can easily deal with excess alkalis if from organic sources. It has great difficulty with inorganic alkalis like iron, calcium, potassium, sodium and magnesium from inorganic sources, that is rocks, ores, soil, metal spring, well waters and cooked foods, especially sea water and cooked foods.

The body has a very difficult time dealing with acidic substances, even if from organic sources! While acid pH minerals like phosphorus, chlorine, sulfur, silicon and bromine are essential in human nutrition, these substances are toxic in the inorganic state. Even within an organic context, they present problems if they predominate over offsetting alkaline pH minerals. When the body digests and processes foods, they are metabolized and have metabolic end products that are either alkaline in pH or acid in pH. Pure water is neutral at 7.0.

The body maintains a hemostatic pH of 7.40. When the pH varies a few points above or below this norm, it suffers either alkalosis or acidosis. Alkalosis usually does not occur if there are excesses of alkaline minerals from organic sources. But, if metabolic end-products are acidic, the body has difficulty dealing with them.

The first order of business for the body that has acidic end-products is to neutralize and expel them from the vital domain lest they cause acidosis. When we eat foods that are acidic in their metabolic end-products, the body neutralizes them with alkalis from its reserves. If we eat meal after meal that consists of mostly acid-forming substances after metabolism, the body exhausts its alkaline reserves and must rob its bones of their alkaline minerals, primarily calcium, in order to neutralize the acid end products. That gives rise to osteoporosis and osteomalacia.

How colds are caused

Colds are one of the simplest sicknesses wherein the body withdraws much of its discretionary energies and redirects them to the task of extraordinary elimination of toxins and morbid matters through the mucous membranes of the respiratory tract and sinuses. When the body's cup runneth over, it enters into the G-O phase of the GIGO syndrome. (GIGO is a computer term that is short for "garbage in, garbage out.").

When we eat cooked foods we take in deranged toxic debris that the body cannot cope with ordinarily. When we eat cooked foods, additives, condiments, so-called herbs and take drugs, we become intoxicated with toxic materials. At some point, in order to maintain its integrity and functionality, the body must get the crud out. Colds are one of the many ways in which the body cleanses itself extraordinarily of internal filth.

How asthma is caused

Asthma can be equated with a cold except that the body eliminates its garbage through the bronchi, thus causing their inflammation and swelling which chokes off respiration.

How most diseases are caused

Most illnesses, ailments, maladies, diseases and body problems are occasioned by the body's methodology in eliminating debris relative to its diathesis (disposition) and vitality. Because all illnesses cumulatively reduce body vitality, bad practices eventually escalate into chronic problems which become degenerative and deadly.

How indigestion, acid stomach and gas emissions are caused

There are a multitude of factors that can contribute to upset stomach, sour stomach, heartburn, belching, foul gas emissions and other intestinal problems. The foremost causes are:

1. Eating foods in combinations that are incompatible in digestive chemistry. This tops the list. Eliminating undigested foods wastes our energies. Besides this, undigested foods do not provide nourishment. Instead, they are fermented, putrefied or made rancid by our intestinal flora. These processes give rise to foul emissions of methane gas, sour stomach, heartburn, etc. and contribute toxic by-products that cause headaches and other pathologies. Fermentation products of bacteria include highly toxic alcohol and acetic acid (vinegar).

2. Eating "foods" that humans are not equipped to digest easily and efficiently. Our natural bacterial population has a field day on indigestible bits of foods.

3. Eating foods with differing digestive times, thus causing the fast-digesting food to be held up so that it ferments or sours. Eating desserts, even fruits, after a regular meal guarantees fermentation.

4. Eating foods that are acid-forming in metabolic reaction. This acidifies the intestinal tract, causing acidosis of the body and

osteoporosis of bones and teeth. The body robs the bones and teeth of alkaline elements to neutralize the acids. This also gives rise to intestinal distress and gas eructations.

5. Eating beyond digestive capacity or overeating. Food eaten beyond digestive capacity causes bacterial fermentation, putrefaction and rancidity, adding up to a grand case of upset stomach.

6. Eating when digestive ability is low, as when one is emotionally upset, under tension or stress, feeling poorly, needing sleep and rest, etc.

7. Eating foods that contain condiments, preservatives, irritants, heated oils, or other toxic substances (e.g., uric acid of meat), etc. Vinegar, e.g., will retard or totally suspend digestion.

8. Eating cooked foods. Cooked cabbage, for instance, takes twice as long in the stomach as raw cabbage.

6
How to Determine Your Natural Dietetic Character

The purpose of this chapter is to ascertain the criteria by which each of us can unerringly ascertain our correct diet. This explorative study, therefore, endeavors to present in incontrovertible, self-evident statements by which such a determination can be made. Of course, we leave no doubt about the determination with our own conclusions and statements. Humans, like every other species in nature, have their natural diet. Just as all species in nature are sensually, aesthetically, psychologically, structurally and physiologically adapted to seek, find, acquire, consume, process and assimilate foods of their dietary character. When nutrient and food requirements of humans have been explored, the criteria point unmistakably to the foods consonant with our dietary disposition. Please consider these big ideas:

1. That we humans developed in nature and, like all creatures that developed in nature, we are specialized and equipped in all aspects of our being to easily discover, acquire, appropriate, digest, absorb and utilize foods to which we are biologically adapted.

2. All acts and practices that humans must do to thrive healthily are pleasurable, delightful and joyful. All acts and practices that entail discomforts and suffering, sickness and pain are unhealthy and a drain upon the organism.

3. Our natural foods have no poisons nor do they, except under very abnormal conditions, lead to our poisoning.

4. Foods contrary to our biological disposition cause our debility, derange our functions, and cause suffering, sickness and disease.

5. Animals and humans in nature that can no longer obtain foods of their dietary disposition suffer famine and starvation. Few can, as humans do, pervert themselves dietarily to survive. Those who pervert there diets suffer grievous diseases as a result.

Some outstanding facts for your consideration

1. While in a state of nature, humans and as well other species developed natural equipment and faculties for finding, taking, consuming, efficiently processing and utilizing foods which they adapted to.

2. Despite the many and varied diets consumed by humans over the globe, our instinctual dietary nature and faculties has not evolved away from our pristine foods.

3. The foods upon which we developed in nature necessarily nourished us adequately to bring us to our high state of development. The foods to which we adapted in nature will still sustain us adequately and amply by meeting all our varied nutrient requirements.

4. With our modern botanical and horticultural expertise, we are capable of producing our natural foods of a quality that will continue to meet our nutrient needs and enable us to attain our highest potentials.

5. Symbiosis and cooperation exist in nature to an extent we do not realize. Certainly our educational media and texts do not teach our symbiotic role in nature. Humans existed symbiotically in nature.

Key words and terms explained

ACID-FORMING: For our purposes, foods which, when metabolized, form acidic end-products. Acids must be neutralized because the body must maintain an alkaline disposition of blood and fluids. Phosphorus, chlorine, sulfur and silicon are the most prevalent acid-forming elements.

AESTHETIC: Relating to beauty or that which is consonant with human well-being. As we use it we mean our sense of beauty.

That which is promotive of human well-being is usually beautiful, and that which is contrary to human well-being is usually ugly and repulsive.

ALKALINE-FORMING: Foods which, when metabolized, form bases or alkalis in the body. Alkalis are base elements that predominate in the body. We require an alkaline disposition of blood and fluids. Calcium, magnesium, sodium, potassium and iron are the most significant alkaline elements.

ALKALOSIS: A body condition wherein acidic minerals are not sufficient to maintain the normal homeostatic pH. A normal bodily pH is in the range of 7.35 to 7.45 (slightly alkaline). When the body becomes overly alkaline, usually due to an overload of inorganic alkalis which the body handles poorly, it experiences distress, some of it being akin to heartburn.

ASSIMILATION: The incorporation of nutrients into body substance or into substances the body needs in its processes and functions.

CARNIVORE: An eater of animals or carnage. Be it noted that carnivores not only eat the flesh of animals but blood, bone, gristle and offal as well. Eating flesh only is a very unbalanced diet.

CONSONANT: Meaning "in accord with," or "in harmony with." As we use it, the term means *in agreement with.*

ENDOGENOUS: Meaning internally originating or generated.

ESSENTIAL FATTY ACIDS: These are the fatty acids occurring within oils and foods which are deemed necessary in the human diet because of human inability to synthesize them. They include linoleic acid, linolenic acid, and arachidonic acid. Evidence has surfaced that now says there may be only one essential fatty acid inasmuch as the body does seem to have the ability to synthesize arachidonic and linolenic acids. Simple fatty acids of all kinds are called monoglycerides.

EXOGENOUS: Something originating outside the organism. For our purposes too, the intestinal tract is outside the organism, being a tube that traverses the body from mouth to anus. Nevertheless, we regard this as internal. Because of this "exogenous" nature of an internal organ (the intestinal tract) this may lead to confusion at times.

FACULTIES: As we use it this means all the resources and equipment an organism possesses for its life activities and processes.

FAMINE: A paucity or shortage of needs or even their total absence. More particularly this applies to occasions of food scarcity or absence.

FRUGIVORE: Animals or humans who live on fruits. For our purposes anyone who lives predominantly or mostly on fruits. There are total fruitarians but they comprise only a fraction of the fruitarians.

FRUIT: That part of a seed package developed and grown specifically by a plant (stalk, vine or tree) to induce consumption with the incidental benefit of the spreading of its seed. Fruit is the only form of plant life grown specifically as food.

GRAMINIVORE: Creatures that subsist on grains and/or cereals. Mostly these are birds. Technically, any creatures that live on grasses and their seeds are graminivorous. But these are generally referred to as herbivores if they consume grasses or other herbage.

HERBIVORE: Eaters of plants which, practically, means mostly grasses, though there are leaf eaters (e.g., giraffes), wood eaters and weed eaters.

INSECTIVORE: A mammalian eater of insects as a primary source of sustenance. These are moles, armadillos, etc.

METABOLIC: Relating to body processes that change substances. There are tearing-down processes called catabolic and building-up processes called anabolic.

MINERAL SALTS: Mineral salts are formed by an organic combination of a mineral with an acid to form a stable compound. This compound can then be metabolized and utilized by the body.

PALATE: Pertaining to the senses of taste. A food is said to be palatable if it appeals to our tastes.

PATHOGENIC: A combination of the Greek words *patho-* which means disease or suffering and *gen* which means to produce. Hence *pathogenic* means that which produces disease.

PERVERTED: Deviant from normal; unnatural; abnormal; wrong action; incorrect.

PHYSIOLOGICAL: Pertaining to the internal processes, functions and activities that attend living organisms. Physiology as such also involves a study of the components and faculties of organisms in connection with processes, functions and activities they're involved in.

PRISTINE: Belonging to a beginning period. An original condition.

PROTEIN: Nitrogenous compounds as organized into amino acids which act as an alphabet from which the body creates over 100,000 words (proteins). These combinations serve as building materials, enzyme catalysts of metabolic activities, and factor in about every bodily process in some way. Proteins are in all living organisms, plant or animal. Every living cell of every living thing is endowed with proteins that have been specially synthesized to meet its special needs. All organisms reject, destroy and expel proteins not of its own synthesis.

RATIONALE: The setting forth of controlling principles or the principles that appertain to a situation. An explanation of why for, what for, how for, etc.

RESERVE: That which is stored in anticipation of future need.

SALIENT: That which is foremost, conspicuous or standing out as we use it.

STARVATION: As we use it, a stage when all fat reserves have been exhausted and the body begins consumption of muscular or proteinaceous tissues for the energies necessary to conduct brain, heart and other vital activities.

SYMBIOSIS: Dissimilar organisms that cooperate for the benefit of both. The cooperation is usually instinctual. A good example is the services rendered flowers by bees and insects in incidentally effecting fertilization while sustaining themselves upon nectar created by the plant to attract their consumption.

SYMBIONT: A participant in symbiotic activities.

SYMBIOTIC: Meaning organisms and/or plants that cooperate with each other or perform services for each other for mutual benefit.

TANTALIZE: That which entices, enthralls or attracts. This means something that entrances us but is out of reach or unavailable. We use this term as that which arouses desire such that we're attracted to it.

TOXIC: Poisonous; anti-vital; relating to a substance that interferes with, impedes, impairs or destroys vital functions and processes due to chemical unions that derange stable processes; that which disturbs homeostasis; that which clogs, blocks or modifies body processes; and that which injures due to its presence or its modifications of the norm.

VEGETARIAN: The word derives from *vegetus* meaning lively, exciting or animated. The word is popularly used to mean an eater of fruits, vegetables, grains, legumes, nuts, seeds and non-animal fare generally. It does not mean, as commonly supposed, an eater of only vegetable fare. On the other hand, we must respect common understanding and usage by regarding the term *vegetarian* as meaning only a consumer of plant foods.

VITAMIN: Means "vital amine," or a coenzyme necessary to metabolic processes. Most vitamins are composed of various amino acid combinations or proteins. Vitamins are under the control of the body in both their composition and employment.

Exogenous and aesthetic requirements of our natural foods

This concerns the properties foods must have to meet the human biological disposition. Needless to say, within the bounds of our concept, our natural foods self-evidently existed in nature sufficiently to supply the needs of the populace of the time. They had to be available in plenitude, otherwise adaptations would not have occurred that we can easily determine. In plenitude of its natural foods, a species thrives and increases in numbers. In scarcity a species suffers famine and, sometimes, starvation within the area affected. Humans normally have reserves sufficient to carry them through famines for 50 to 60 days. Almost all species have adaptations that enable them to survive deprivation for periods of time.

Aesthetic requirements of our natural foods

To have been a natural food for humans, their needs must have been met for a period sufficiently long to have occasioned the development of equipment and faculties that appreciated it, and that surely and efficiently apprehended, acquired, consumed, digested, absorbed and utilized it.

Our natural foods, therefore, must arouse our attention and desires as they exist or existed in nature. To attract our attention as foods, our natural foods must be beautiful to the human eye. Our sense of beauty revolves around that which is consonant with our well-being. This is called our aesthetic disposition. This sense developed and became fixed by experience interacting with and modified by that which yielded value, that which was endowed with the qualities that repeatedly gratified and supplied our physiological needs.

1. *A natural food must appeal to the eye.* The first requisite of a natural food is that it must attract the eye in its natural state. Our eyes are our foremost organs of discovery. Experience and instinct must fix a recognition of the food as desirable.

2. *A natural food must tantalize the sense of smell.* To be a natural food it must be redolent, aromatic or fragrant enough to arouse desire in those that smell it with their olfactory senses.

3. *A natural food must be easy to apprehend and acquire with our natural faculties.* The third requisite of a natural food is ease of discovery and acquisition with our natural faculties. With our eyes, sense of smell, physical faculties, especially our legs, feet, arms and hands, we must be able to acquire quantities sufficient to meet our needs within our diurnal time frame.

Our natural foods must be easily consumed in their natural state as modified by our natural faculties only

Foods of our biological and symbiotic nature are not always

ready to consume. After acquisition they usually require some external processing in order that their nutrients be easily bitten off, chewed and swallowed. Humans are the most fastidious of all eaters on earth, rivaled perhaps only by other primates such as the chimp, orangutan and gorilla.

External food processing for humans means we must prepare the food for mouth by peeling off skins, cracking of shells, and otherwise exposing the food portion to the teeth such that bite-sized morsels may be facilitated.

Our natural foods must be a gustatory delight in their natural state

Humans lived for millennia in nature before they became tool users and mastered fire. Tools do not occasion evolvement, but rather the fixation of existing faculties. Therefore any food, to be natural, must excite our palate and be delightful in the natural unfired state. The eating of a natural food must be a cherished and palate ravishing experience, as all acts necessary to our well-being are blissful.

Endogenous requirements of our natural foods

Our natural foods are the raw materials the body's internal faculties use to meet its requirements. Our natural foods must be replete with our nutrient needs and contain no components which devitalize or poison the body.

Our natural foods will not intoxicate or poison us!

The first commandment of eating is: "Thou shalt not poison thyself." The average American commits from 10 to 80 poisonings acts daily. Our natural foods contain only components which have inherent enzymes that break them down into their basic nutrients or simplest forms. Our natural foods require almost no enzyme secretion from our secretory faculties for basic digestion. If a food has components or compounds for which we secrete no digestive enzymes, that component is toxic to our bodies and occasions considerable distress to most. Such components or compounds are of-

42

ten referred to as "allergens." A natural food has no "allergens" at all though some of us may be abnormally sensitive to biologically correct foods. The foremost "allergens" are really proper body objection to toxic substances or substances that its faculties cannot digest. Poisons the average American consumes consist not only of recreational drugs, but of foods ingested with toxic components or which, in the course of intestinal transit, are bacterially and/or fungally transformed into toxic putrefactive and/or fermentative products.

Our natural foods must be easily and efficiently digested and utilized

Animals in nature are equipped to easily and efficiently handle their natural foods. This is true of humans as well. What other animals may easily digest and assimilate may be impossible for us. We must recognize that many foods are predigested, that is, the enzymes of the foods break themselves down into simple nutrients as needed by their biological symbionts. Predigestion is, of course, the ultimate accommodation between symbionts. The less efficiently the food is digested, the worse it is for you. The more efficiently the food is digested, the better it is for you. Perhaps it can better be expressed this way: More strain, more drain. Less strain, more gain.

Our natural foods must have nutrient adequacy that proportionately supplies our various needs

Food symbiotic to a species amply supplies every nutrient need. This means that it does undersupply or oversupply any of our nutrient requirements to a burdensome or pathological extent. For instance, grass is a complete food for cattle. If foods are not symbiotic with the consuming species, certain nutrient needs must necessarily be met. Failure to meet nutrient needs results in deficiencies. Deficiencies give rise to many problems other than the obvious deficiency.

The RDAs or Recommended Dietary Allowances published by the NRC or Nutritional Research Council is deemed the most authoritative there is in this country, even though it is askew and at considerable variance with requirements established in other countries. The parameters and criteria they observed in the setting of the RDAs are relevant only to conventional living Americans and quite out of line for a healthy person's requirements living on naturally ordained foods. Nevertheless, knowing NRC's guidelines and methodologies gives us ballpark proportions of our nutrient needs.

The RDA for a 154-pound man is 2,700 calories per day for conventional eaters. If 30% of those calories are from fat, which is the maximum the NRC recommends, that means there are roughly 810 fat calories or roughly 90 grams of pure fat or fats in the solid state, thus leaving 1,890 calories to be supplied by proteins and carbohydrates. As the RDA is 56 grams of protein, 224 calories worth (which we really do not use for fuel), this leaves 1,666 calories to come from carbohydrates. That figures out to be about 417 grams of pure carbohydrate. The RDA's for the aggregate amount of mineral matter and vitamins figure out to about 6 grams of solids of the 563 grams of food solids computed above. The RDAs have us consuming, in practice, the following as a percentage or proportion of our diet:

Carbohydrates: *74% by weight of solids, 62% of calories.*

Proteins: *10% by weight of solids, 8% by calories.*

Fats: *16% by weight of solids, 30% by calories.*

Mineral matter: *1% by weight but as a part of the primary nutrients.*

It should be noted that mineral matter is actually a part of the protein, carbohydrate and fat portions and has no separate consideration in the RDAs by weight. Vitamins constitute such a small part of 1% as to have neither weight nor caloric considerations.

As the calories of proteins are for measurement only, there being a greater expenditure of calories in humans in their digestion, deamination and use than is obtained from them, we may not take them into account in the consideration of caloric requirements.

Our natural foods must adequately supply our caloric needs

The RDA for our caloric needs is about 50% too high! Our

natural foods in their natural state yield more usable calories than cooked foods. Thus the caloric needs of an active 154-pound man (70 kilos) per day is really about 1,800 calories per studies by Drs. Alexander Leaf and Mark Hegstead of Harvard University.

As the NRC recommends a maximum of 30% calories from fat, with some of its members even recommending under 10% in this form, you can see that fats have a secondary rating as a nutrient. Our essential fatty acid needs are really only about 1% to 2% of our net nutrient needs by weight according to RDAs and about 2.25% to 4.5% of our caloric needs. Thus, for nutrient considerations, carbohydrate food solids from which we derive calories can be, and perhaps should be, weight-wise, near 90%.

As fiber is a neutral factor, being virtually unused in its passage through the intestinal tract, we need not consider it as a nutrient even though its caloric values are included in conventional figures because it is a firebox calorie. For convenience sake we'll leave our caloric requirements as being weight-wise and calorie-wise about 90% of our utile diet. It is perhaps an accurate figure for natural food eaters.

Our foremost fuel is glucose and fructose. The body can use these as is. If we eat starches we must heat them to dextrinize them, thus facilitating their breakdown into glucose. Our starch-eating license is very limited which indicates it is not a natural food. As glucose and fructose are our natural sugars, there is about 95% energy gain if we get these directly from our foods, whereas an equal amount of energy in raw starches yields perhaps 40% of its potential (humans secrete no enzymes needed to break down the cellular membranes that protect starch globules—all breakdown is due to crushing and chewing), as long as our limited secretion of the starch-splitting enzyme amylase holds out. When heated to the point of dextrinization of the starch, the cellular membranes burst by expansion. Even so, because of the problems involved with cooked fare, the body can realize only 65% to 70% of the energy potential of starchy foods.

Our natural foods must adequately supply our amino acid needs

Note that I have said amino acids because our actual needs are for amino acids, not proteins. If we eat proteins, they must be laboriously digested, that is, broken down by body enzymatic action into amino acids.

Our needs for amino acids are about 21 grams per day, or 84 calories. This is the finding of Dr. Mark Hegstead of Harvard University. The NRC also recognizes 21 grams as the real RDA for amino acids in setting 56 grams as a 154-pound man's needs. They enhanced the 21 grams by 33% and then doubled it as a margin of safety to arrive at the RDA of 56 grams. When you've got your building built, throwing extra bricks into it may jam things up.

Twenty one grams of amino proteins in a diet consisting of about 500 grams of usable nutrient solids required daily is about 4%. In our natural diet the amino acids are about 100% usable whereas in the conventional American diet they are only about 20% usable! The average American consumes about 105 grams of protein daily, but mostly in a cooked form. Cooking coagulates, deranges and deaminates proteins and amino acids, thus rendering them unusable except as carbohydrates. In the cooked and oxidized form they are very readily putrefiable.

Ninety percent of amino acid and protein wastes of the body are recycled. This means that proteins involved in body processes are providentially used and reused. It also means that losses through cellular death are largely reclaimed and reused. The overall loss is thus about 10% of the daily usage. It is estimated that the body of the average man requires about 230 grams of new protein formation daily. If 90% of this is supplied by recycling spent proteins, then only about 23 grams of new protein need to be consumed.

Our natural foods must supply our needs for mineral matter

Mineral matter that the human body uses consists of minerals in an organic context, that is, in a colloidal form within living substance. Heat quickly destroys the organic context, thus returning mineral matter to an inorganic state. Though super fine in consistency, minerals that were in the organic state become, through the agency of heat or decomposition of their medium, inorganic the same as they occur in soil, rocks, ores, etc. In this form they are not utile by the human body except in certain applications. For example, base minerals will alkalinize the intestinal tract even though they cannot be assimilated.

Minerals which the body requires become toxic if appropriated in an inorganic context. This is easily demonstrable. Leukocytosis is recognized as a pathological state. This is a proliferation of white blood cells, the whole of which is often referred to as our immune system. If the components of a cooked or heat-deranged meal are taken, leukocytosis results. If only inorganic minerals are ingested, leukocytosis likewise results. Leukocytosis is a body defensive act wherein the body unleashes huge armies of white blood cells to apprehend and carry toxic substances to the nearest exit or put them harmlessly under the rug somewhere.

Thus the body must have, according to the RDAs, about 1% of its solid food intake as minerals. To be usable these minerals must be in an un-deranged organic state.

Our natural foods must supply our needs for fatty acids

There was, at one time, proclaimed to be three essential fatty acids, namely arachidonic, linoleic and linolenic. Today only linoleic is said by nutritional researchers to be essential. Popularly, linolenic fatty acids are referred to as omega-3 while linoleic fatty acids are referred to as omega-6. Essential means that the body has a need of a component or components, in this case fatty acids, because it cannot itself synthesize them. Our natural foods must, of course, contain our needs for essential fatty acids, because the body never found it necessary to develop faculties to produce them or they were so plentiful in the food the body ceased to produce them and lost its ability to do so as it did with vitamin C and certain amino acids recognized as essential.

Our natural foods must supply our needs for vitamins

While vitamins comprise such a small portion of our total dietary need that all the RDAs taken together on an annual basis could be put into a sewing thimble, they are, nevertheless, essential to our well-being. The RDAs for vitamins vary with each vitamin. Here I will not deal with individual vitamins as separate components. At this time only the observation need be made that our natural foods must adequately contain these vitamins or give rise to them in absorbable form while in the intestinal tract.

Our natural foods must supply our needs for miscellaneous nutrients

The above nutrients are said to be macronutrients though, as can be seen, vitamins are really micronutrients. Other micronutrients which the body may require are auxones (certain plant hormones). The science of nutrition is yet young. Whether or not there are needed nutrients in foods other than the five categories of solids treated above remains open to question.

In any event you can be sure our natural foods are replete with all the nutrients we need in the quantities we require. After all, our virtual abandonment of our natural dietary fare is only a few seconds on the clock if we regard our earthly existence as being 24 hours thus far. And our *natural fare* is scientifically established as responsible for our high state of development.

Our natural foods should supply our water needs

Inasmuch as humans, like many desert creatures, have no natural water drinking equipment, that is, no provision therefor, our natural dietary should be water sufficient just as it is in the case of desert animals as well as numerous other creatures in nature.

Healthy people eating their natural diet usually have a surplus of water without drinking. The addition of some foods without sufficient water, less than 25% water content, does not occasion thirst. However, substances with water content equal to or greater than our natural foods occasion thirst if ingested cooked, if they are biologically incorrect, if they are condimented, especially with salt, and toxic substances in general.

While thirst generally arises from pathogenic conditions within, there are exceptions: extraordinarily warm climatic conditions, extraordinarily low humidity, periods without normal food intake, partaking of good foods that have been dried, heavy labor or exercise under warm conditions, and yet other conditions. When thirst arises, always drink water—pure water. With ready supplies of pure water and tools that facilitate drinking such as cups, glasses, etc., we can easily drink the water necessary to make up deficits.

Our diet must be alkaline, overall, in metabolic end products

Humans require a diet that is alkaline in its metabolic end products. For practical purposes this means at least 80% of alkaline-forming foods against not more than 20% of acid end-product foods. The human homeostatic condition is alkaline with essential fluids normally having a pH of 7.40. Any significant variation in the pH can result in coma and death. Acidosis is deadlier than alkalosis. The body can rather easily discharge excess organic alkalis, but must first neutralize excess acids. In the absence of sufficient alkalis, the body must take alkaline minerals, including calcium, from bones and fluids to effect neutralization. Americans eat a predominantly acid-forming diet, a diet that is not only pathogenic in itself, but causes such complications as base mineral depletion characterized by osteoporosis and metabolic disorders.

What would you eat in nature? Considering various foods and our natural disposition

Despite the gross perversion of our instincts, they are still alive and well and will reassert should we be relegated back to nature. Therefore, this quest is to ascertain what we would eat in nature. Our instinctive foods, the foods which helped to develop us to our magnificence, necessarily contain all that we need to thrive on. This assurance being soundly based, as you will soon determine for yourself, it then behooves us, as responsible members of society, to undertake the course which makes us the most we can be so that we can maximally serve ourselves and those who depend on us. This is a mutual arrangement, as those whom we serve in turn serve us better. This exalts everyone and has a ripple effect that makes all in our society healthier and happier, more loving and more caring. In serving yourself best, you at the same time serve others best. This inquiry will survey almost all the foods that humans, in their varied habits, eat. We'll consider each as a possible food for ourselves as it occurs in nature without benefit of cooking apparati, tools and containers. Remember, your instincts will reject or cherish each food on its merits, that is, its appeals to your senses and palate, the only criteria that guided us to food selection in plentiful nature,

Our premises are: that Mother nature, i.e., the sum of all factors and influences under which we lived in nature, served us correctly to start with, inasmuch as we thrived and attained our high station in its midst; that what was right for us then is still right for us in view that we're still structurally and physiologically the same as we were during most of our sojourn as humans in nature; that we can still, within our modern context, supply ourselves with natural foods substantially and significantly; and that we can also observe, meaningfully, the other requisites of life in our modern context.

Pertinent questions—the answers to which determine our natural diet

Are we herbivores?
Are we graminivores?
Are we root grubbers?
Are we insectivores?
Are we carnivores?
Are we eaters of fermented and rotten foods?
Are we sucklings of animals?
Are we frugivores?
Are we vegetarians?
Are we nut and seed eaters?

Are we fat eaters?

Are we protein eaters?

Are we starch eaters?

Are we all the foregoing, that is, omnivores?

Are we herbivores?

Herbivores are natural consumers of herbage such as grass, weeds, leaves, stalks and stems. Does foraging in nature for grass, weeds and leaves appeal to you? Do grass and weeds attract your eye, tantalize your sense of smell and excite your palate?

Of course it is repulsive to you for the very simple reason that it cannot satisfy your needs. You do not secrete cellulase or other enzymes that break down these plants as herbivores do. Therefore you cannot derive your foremost need from them, namely simple sugars which is your body's primary fuel. Rather, the processing and problems caused by their ingestion occasion *a net loss of energies*.

Of course, humans do consume some herbage such as lettuce, celery, cabbage family members, (kale, cabbage, collards, Brussels sprouts, cauliflower, broccoli, bok choy, etc.), spinach and yet other leafy greens. Plain, as they occur in nature, these vegetables really do not appeal to us though we can cultivate (pervert) a taste for much of it. At least cauliflower and broccoli do yield some calories and all yield, to the extent when digested, proteins, some essential fatty acids, mineral matter and vitamins. But, if we get enough of these nutrients from our natural foods, then these are not needed from plants that we do not eat raw with keen relish.

If we had to rely on herbage exclusively for our foods, we'd adjust somewhat but, in all likelihood, slowly starve as the calorie yield is negative or very low. While cooking destroys most of the abundant nutrients, it also converts the cellulose, fibers and other components into usable caloric values.

Let's face it! Though we will include vegetables in our dietary, we're not vegetable eaters by nature. *Obviously we're not herbivores.*

Are we graminivores?

Being graminivorous means we live from grasses and grass seeds though grass eaters are really called herbivores. Strict grain eaters are called graminivores. Many birds in nature live on grass and weed seeds. Grass seeds include wheat, oats, rye, barley and rice which were developed by human mastery of nature only within the last 10,000 years. There are thousands of other grass seeds that occur throughout nature.

Of course, we'd all reject grass seeds as items of diet in nature. First, they are in a condition we can neither masticate nor digest. Being heavy on starches, we would gag on the equivalent of a spoonful or two. You might try a mouthful of wheat berries without husks removed as you must eat them in nature. Won't work for us. Further, if you ate a tablespoon of raw flour made from grass seeds (cereal grains), you'd gag.

As grass seeds neither attract, tantalize nor arouse us in their raw natural state, we can reject them as natural human fare even though most of the human race presently consumes grains. Thus, we are not natural graminivores.

Are we natural root grubbers?

Animals that naturally grub for roots have snouts. As most roots are starchy, root grubbers secrete a plethora of starch-splitting enzymes whereas humans secrete only one such enzyme, amylase, in very limited quantities. Humans abhor dirt, are quite fastidious and refuse to eat anything dirt covered or even dirt tinged. Hogs and grubbers pass lots of dirt through their bodies. Without tools humans are very poor diggers. They have no motivation to do so for there are no foods below ground that, in their natural state, please the palate. Humans can handle very little that comes out of the ground in its raw natural state. Some roots, notably turnips, rutabagas, sweet potatoes, yams, ground nuts, beets, carrots, parsnips and salsify can be eaten raw. In practice today, practically none are eaten raw. In nature we would be obligated to do without tools and would have to eat them raw or not at all. In our natural habitat of plenitude, we can be sure that roots which man could handle without tools received precious little attention as food.

In view of the considerations, you can write off humans as natural root grubbers and I'm sure you'll concur.

Are we insectivores?

There are humans who eat insects, especially grasshoppers and ants. But, by and large, humans would give insects a big "yuk" when it comes to eating them, especially in the raw state. For the gourmands who eat them, they must fry them in batter or chocolate coat them, a way of saying they are not delicious fare in themselves. There are many birds that live exclusively on insects when and where they are plentiful. There are bats which live on insects. But I know of no humans who do.

The average person is repulsed by insects rather than attracted to them as yummy foods. I don't relish them raw or cooked and I don't think you do either.

Are we carnivores?

A carnivore is an eater of carnage or flesh. This does not accurately portray animals said to be carnivores. Animals that live on other animals usually consume most of the animal, not merely the flesh. True carnivores lap the flowing and oozing blood of their prey with relish. They delight in the guts and its partially digested contents. And they will consume the bones and gristle (collagen or cartilage). Dogs, for instance, require about 1,700% as much calcium as humans, for animal flesh is extremely acid-forming. Blood and bones are required to offset the acidotic end materials. They also require about 1,200% more protein than humans. When you note the relish and gusto with which dogs go for whole animals, you can be sure that what carnivores need for their nourishment is quite delicious to them.

Do you relish the idea of crushing the life of a rabbit with your bare hands and teeth? Can you lick its blood with gusto, getting it over your face, hands and body? Would you dig into its guts with pleasure? Would you love to chew on its bones and gristle? Would you love to swallow chunks of its flesh, not being fastidious about swallowing hair and vermin that might be involved? Would you like to do the same for any plant-eating animal that you could apprehend, kill and consume while still in its warm and fresh state?

Of course, you and every unperverted person loves animals as fellow creatures on earth. Killing them is repulsive to you and eating them in the freshly killed state is even more disgusting to you. Yet, most of us do consume flesh and some organ meats while rejecting blood, bone, most fats and the entrails or offal. But we kill our animals by proxy. We denature and derange flesh and organs with heat and camouflage it with condiments. Does this describe a carnivore to you? Would you, in a state of nature, relish chasing down animals and eating them? Again, this is alien to your natural disposition and actually sickening.

True carnivores also secrete an enzyme called uricase to metabolize the some 5% uric acid in flesh. We secrete none and thusly must neutralize it with our alkaline minerals, primarily calcium. The resulting calcium urate crystals are one of the many pathogens of meat-eating, in this case giving rise to or contributing to gout, arthritis, rheumatism and bursitis.

Are humans natural meat-eaters? There are too many considerations in physiology, structure (miscalled anatomy), aesthetic disposition and psychology that characterize us as nonflesh eaters to even seriously entertain such notions.

I had a nutritionist tell me in front of an audience that we had canine teeth and that proved our meat-eating character. I responded with: "You really mean dog teeth, don't you? Like fangs?" This caused her to redden. Then I related one of Abraham Lincoln's favorite retorts: "If you counted a sheep's tail as a leg, how many legs would it have?" Invariably the answer was "five." To which Lincoln would respond: "Only four. Counting the tail as a leg doesn't make it one."

I think you'll agree that we are not equipped in any aspect of our being as carnivores.

Are we eaters of fermented and rotten foods?

Substantially all of Americans eat fermented and putrefied substances that are called foods. When fats oxidize and decompose they become rancid and repulsive. Carbohydrates ferment when decomposed by fungi (yeast) and bacteria. And proteins putrefy (rot) when decomposed by bacteria and fungi.

It is odd that we will discard fermented grapes, yet drink their fermentation end product called wine. Odder still, most Americans consume with relish something that never occurred in nature, a pathogenic putrefactive product called cheese. Cheese represents about all the decomposition products in a single package: rancid fats, putrefactive products and fermentation products.

Bacterial and fungal (yeast) fermentation produce alcohol, vinegar (acetic acid) and lactic acid with other by-products of methane and carbon dioxide. Proteins, decomposed primarily by anaerobic bacteria but also by fungi and aerobic bacteria, have as decomposition end products ptomaines (putrescine, muscarine, neurine, cadaverine, ptomatropine and yet other toxic compounds), indoles, leukomaines, skatoles, mercaptans, ammonia, methane, hydrogen sulfide and yet other toxic compounds. You need only to refer to a good dictionary to learn just how poisonous these products are. Yet, Americans eat billions upon billions of pounds of cheese annually.

Cheese is made by taking the casein portion of milk and rotting it with types of bacteria that yield by-products that many palates have come to treasure. That all these poisons going into the system cause anything less than sicknesses, diseases and debility is misrepresentation. Tumors and cancer are often the result.

Humans consume many fermentation, rancid and putrefactive products. Most are derived from milk. Some are derived from grains (especially the alcohols), fruits (wines and certain vinegars), legumes (especially the soy bean and its train of putrefactive products), and decomposed meats.

As humans could not consume these decomposed products in nature without tools and containerization, we may safely categorize them as unnatural. I dare say that you agree.

Are we sucklings of animals?

I doubt that humans ever directly suckled cattle, goats, mares, camels, sheep and other animals. And, of course, the idea of doing this is obnoxious to our disposition. I refer, facetiously, to milk eaters as secondhand grass eaters although, to be sure, grass has all the nutrients necessary to support life.

While we can live on milks (certain Africans like the Masai live substantially on milk and blood, thus reducing themselves to parasite status), these are by no means our natural foods. Milk-drinking as a regular part of our intake is only a few hundred years old with the exception of certain Arabic and African peoples. Milk-drinking is pathogenic. If milk and milk products were discontinued today, millions of people would cease to suffer sicknesses and pathologies within a short period. In fact, if this alone was discontinued, the hospitals would virtually empty out and physicians' waiting rooms would be mostly vacated.

Milk-drinking is also an act by proxy. If we had to get milk directly from the teats of animals by suction, I'm sure we'd skirt milk altogether. I would and I'm sure you would too.

Are we frugivores?

Are we a species of fruit-eaters? Would you, in nature, relish ripe grapes, peaches, melons, bananas, apples, plums, oranges, mangos, avocados, tomatoes, figs, berries and the thousands of other fruits? Would fruits attract your eye, tantalize your sense of smell, and be a gustatory delight in their raw natural ripe state? Would you prefer anything that occurs in nature to a juicy sweet watermelon?

Man has always had a love affair going with fruits. Even through all his perversions, he has continued to relish fruits. Fruits are the natural food of humans and the only food category ideally suited to all their faculties. This does not mean we should eat fruits totally and exclusively in our present circumstances, but it does mean that, in nature, that's all we ate as attested to by anthropological evidence scientists have uncovered, notably Dr. Alan Walker of Johns

Hopkins University.

Of course, you go for fruits in their raw state regardless of what else your acculturization and circumstances dispose you to eat. Your instincts are still alive and well despite perversions. Many myths have been built around and about fruits. As a fruitarian I can offer a new dietary for those who say we're not—their own words!

Nutritionists, so-called, are the creatures of training dictated by the meat, grain and milk trusts. These trusts are part of the dominant commercial interests that dictate what will be taught in our educational institutions from universities down to kindergarten. Nutritionists are trained like seals to parrot the propaganda which will induce the populace to consume their masters' products, with the basic five food groups being one of the primary propaganda weapons put at their disposal to serve their masters. Of course, there are renegade nutritionists and dietitians who have revolted against the basic four except for the fruit and vegetable category. Most nutritionists are ashamed of the fifth food category and don't even mention it though it is on the books along with the basic four.

The fifth category consists of what might broadly be termed "accessory foods" such as oils, syrups, snack foods, sugars, wines, seasonings, jams, preserves, etc. Even though we are admonished to eat from all five food categories daily by the framers of this scheme to peddle commercial products, nutritionists and dietitians are not keen on mouthing this part of the propaganda even though they include it liberally in their recipes.

While some nutritionists and dietitians praise fruits and vegetables, they still characterize those who point out our biologically correct foods as faddists and nutritional quacks. Yet, even in seminars, those who sharply question me must admit that, aesthetically, they would eat little besides fruits in nature and that we humans are naturally fruitarians.

All the criteria heretofore cited as the requirements of our natural foods are amply met by fruits. In short, they are replete with our nutrient requirements in practically the proportions that we need them. We are biological symbionts of fruit-bearing plants, and in nature would eat very little besides fruits. Despite all this, there's no particular harm in eating green leafy vegetables, stalks, stems and their fresh juices in the raw state. Even some steaming or conservative cooking of tubers, stalks, stems, roots, corms and selected legumes and grains (preferably sprouted), are not sufficiently deleterious to seriously harm our health. Of course, there are some toxic results from eating all this fare. We're better off without them. Yet, I repeat, there is no great harm in their consumption relative to what is suffered from conventional fare.

Dr. Bruce Ames of the University of California, Berkeley, has created a catalog of poisons in vegetables and published an extensive article in the September 23, 1983 issue of *Science* magazine. No indictment of fruits as having toxic substances was made or can be made. Virtually every vegetable was indicted. All were a part of the same study. Humans are biologically equipped to handle most fruits.

When ripened, fruits accommodatingly convert their carbohydrate components into glucose and fructose, simple sugars we can use without further digestion. Their enzymes convert their proteins into amino acids and their fats into fatty acids and glycerols. Thus, when we eat fruits, all we need do is savor their goodness. The fruit portions, that is, mesocarps, were specifically compounded to attract biological symbionts. Fruits meet their nutrient needs rather ideally with predigested nutrients. For humans, no other food compares with fruits in satisfying all needs including, of course, our requirement for delicious soul-exalting fare.

I'm sure that you will agree through your own senses that fruits would be your primary food in a state of nature.

Are we vegetarian?

The average American understands the term vegetarian to mean an "eater of vegetables." But, in reality a vegetarian is someone who eats only plant-derived foods. This may include a preponderance of fruits but, in practice, it means anything and everything besides animal products.

The word vegetable derives from the Latin vegetus meaning lively, exciting or animated. It does not mean specific types of foods other than those which enliven or sustain us in an energetic mode. Necessarily, by this definition, fruits are high energy foods whereas vegetables are either low energy foods or have drawbacks. Typical present-day vegetarian fare includes grains, tubers, root, stalks, stems, leaves, nuts, seeds, fruits, legumes and about everything else that does not move, bleed, cry or resist acquisition.

Even though those who eat all fruits or a preponderance of them can correctly be called fruitarians, they may also be correctly called vegetarians. Personally, my intake is mostly fruit. I prefer to be called a fruitarian, though I do not object to being called a vegetarian. Do you agree that, naturally, we are fruit eaters?

Are we nut and seed eaters?

In nature there is no doubt but that humans did consume some nuts. Even so, our ability to derive nuts from their hard shells is limited. We do not have razor sharp teeth and tons of pressure per bite or jaw-power as have squirrels. Humans can crack certain nuts with their teeth. Very few of today's degenerated version of humans can do it, but most nuts can be cracked with strong jaws and good teeth. Even strong hands can crush nuts if at least two are taken and pressed against each other.

Most nuts are delicious to us in their raw state. Unfortunately, our ability to handle nuts is rather poor. Nuts that we savor are in a storage form, that is, as fats, proteins and invert sugars or starches. Digestion of nuts into fatty acids, amino acids, and glucose is a long drawn out process, most often taking hours. Whether we did or did not consume nuts in nature makes little difference to us to-day. Most of us do consume nuts but disadvantageously as cooked fare. Heated fats and proteins are quite pathogenic, yes, even carcinogenic. Nuts should be eaten raw or not at all.

Technically and botanically nuts are fruits. I do not buy that because the word fruit really means product or result. Fruits are really the mesocarps of seed packages which plants created specifically as a product to be consumed by a biological symbiont who would incidentally discard and distribute the seeds. Nuts and seeds were created by plants for broadcast and reproduction by other methods. All nuts are seeds. Most seeds are in a storage form to survive the vagaries of climatic and consuming elements so that they may be instrumental in reproducing and perpetuating their kind. Nuts, however, have extra protection in that they have hard woody shells. Seeds usually have only fibrous coatings as their protection. Both seeds and nuts are heavily endowed with nutrients sufficient to initiate and sustain a certain minimum growth of their plants. We can benefit from these nutrients. But if we eat more than two or three ounces, we're likely to get more protein and fats than we can readily handle.

Certainly nuts and seeds were not created by plants for consumption but, rather, for reproduction. That some animals have adapted to their consumption has not been a two-sided affair as it has been with fruits where the love affair has been and still is mutual. There are many types of seeds: legumes, grains, weeds, nuts, and fruit seeds being among the most prominent. In their natural state humans can handle very few of these seeds. Nuts can be digested and used in very small amounts. Likewise, sesame, pumpkin, squash, sunflower, pignolias, and some other seeds can be used.

We are primarily carbohydrate eaters, not fat and protein eaters. I dare say you agree with my assessment of nuts and seeds as human fare.

Are we fat eaters?

In nature there are very few fats we can get in any quantity without violating our biological disposition. Avocados, durians, olives, coconuts, nuts and seeds are heavy on fats. Avocados and durians furnish fats in a predigested state when ripe. Coconuts furnish fats as monoglycerides/glycerols before they set their fats as triglycerides in a storage form. Coconuts are, therefore, in the jelly-like state, easily digested. When matured and hardened, it is almost impossible to digest them.

Broccoli and cauliflower have considerable fatty acids in an easily usable state when eaten in the raw fresh condition. However, they give some unwanted toxic sulfur compounds. We get predigested fats adequate to meet our fatty acid needs from fruits. An occasional avocado or seeds and nuts are quite satisfying. Those who subsist substantially on fats do not do well. Eskimos are very short-lived. They consume about 200 grams, about 1,800 calories, daily. Their short-lived condition is probably more attributable to their heavy protein consumption than fats. They consume about 200 grams of protein daily incidental to their fat-eating and this places a great burden upon their organs, especially liver and kidneys. Because of the acid-forming properties of metabolized proteins, Eskimos lose their teeth at an early age and suffer severe osteoporosis. Eskimos are eaters of animal fats and proteins, primarily as derived from fish. Be it noted that, during the berry picking season, Eskimos are said to eat only berries during the short season they are ripening.

Biologically we are not a species of fat eaters, but incidental eaters of fats. Fruits that have lots of fat are predigested so that we handle them with ease when they are ripe. Other forms of fat require hours for their digestion, quite atypical of fruits to which we are most favorably disposed. Fats may lie in the small intestine several hours before bile is secreted into it with which to emulsify them, thus exposing them to lipases which reduce them to monoglycerides (fatty acids) and glycerols.

I adjudge that we are not a species of fat eaters except incidental to our fruitarian disposition.

Are we protein eaters?

To hear the exponents of the meat trust, you'd think we're in imminent danger of disease and death if we fail to eat meat three times a day. The truth is that eating meat three times daily will cause the very conditions we're taught to fear. We're in no danger of protein deficiency unless we're eating a 100% cooked food diet. On the other hand, there are grave dangers in eating cooked proteins. At normal cooking temperatures, proteins are coagulated, deaminated and largely oxidized. The nitrogenous materials are soil for putrefactive bacteria. The carbohydrate portions of cooked proteins are usable for caloric values but still present the problems that cooked carbohydrates pose.

If we must eat proteins, we must eat them raw to derive their full benefit. But proteins, per se, are not created as food. They are created by plant and animal life as components of organisms, seeds, enzymes, ova, etc. Most proteins of this nature have toxic protective compounds. The bean family have anti-enzyme factors. Eggs have avidin. Nuts also have anti-enzyme factors. Seeds of peaches, apples and many other fruits have hydrocyanide. Humans do not secrete the enzymes to negate or break down these toxic substances.

From fruits we derive as much protein as is present in mother's milk for a growing baby! Moreover, fruit proteins come to us predigested as do other ripened fruit components. There are many alarmists who warn us about protein deficiencies of fruits and many other presumed deficiencies. If we developed in nature on fruits to our high state as anthropologists have found, then the real deficiencies are in the thinking of those who proclaim deficiencies. Their evidence is usually based on researches with pathological specimens, especially those whose metabolic and assimilative faculties are very impaired. They base their thinking from a standpoint of disease rather than health, from a modality and curing mentality rather than a correction of pathogenic practices. In saying that our natural foods are deficient, they are simultaneously proclaiming improvidence in nature. Or, in effect, saying: "God, you made a terrible mistake in providing for us and especially in giving us a sweet tooth." Advocating the consumption of proteins and yet more proteins when those so advising know by their own researches and knowledge that the proteins will be cooked and contribute to heavy pathology is nothing less than criminal.

One more consideration: If we ate only proteins in their raw state we'd quickly become diseased and perhaps even suffer death! Why? Because various amino acids require from about 60% to

137% of their carbohydrate energy potential for their deamination and utilization. The net result would be starvation. That's one reason so much weight is lost by the obese on protein diets. And the intoxication that results from putrefaction is the reason so many of these dieters become diseased with some dying.

Are we protein eaters? Emphatically, no!

Are we starch eaters?

To test this question I will not ask you to do the impossible, i.e., take a hand full of grass seeds (presuming you could gather them in nature) and start chewing. Or, try a spoonful of flour of any grain. You'd choke up on the first spoon of it as your starch license (salivary amylase) would be speedily exhausted. This would amply prove to you that we were not starch eaters in nature when we had not mastered fire. Instead of being a palate tingling delight, starches are a torturesome affair.

When humans can freely eat starchy roots, grains and tubers such as cassava, taro, potatoes and wheat in their raw state to satiation and proclaim the experience a gourmet treat, then both you and I might accede that we're starch eaters.

Are we omnivores, that is, all of the foregoing?

Of course, humans are omnivores in practice with the aid of condiments, taste excitants, denaturalization by cooking, camouflaging seasonings, spices and so on. But, in nature, we could not do more than eat foods in season, and we'd have to eat them in the raw state on their own merits with our taste buds. In nature we were frugivores only.

* * *

Humans & Fruit: Symbiotic Partners in Life

While few biology books proclaim symbiosis and none that I've encountered proclaim our own symbiotic role in nature, we are symbionts as are thousands of species. Symbiosis is cooperation between dissimilar organisms for mutual benefit. Symbionts are cooperators in symbiotic living. While the word symbiont is supposed to apply only to the lesser of two cooperating organisms, I prefer to call both of the complementary cooperators symbionts for that is the only nomenclature that makes sense. Let us observe this phenomenon in nature.

We see flowers bloom and put forth tons upon tons of pollen for fertilizing the ovaries of female flowers. Both male and female flowers secrete nectar at their inner base to attract consumption by bees and other insects. In taking such a large reward the bees and insects become contaminated with pollen in the male flowers only to have it removed when they take the nectar of female flowers. The ovaries of female flowers secrete a sticky substance which the bee or insect must come in contact with in taking their nectars. Instances of symbiosis abound in nature.

The above is cited to demonstrate natural cooperativeness or symbiosis. In this case we see that the flowers of plants, both woody and nonwoody, attracted bees and insects to take the free meals provided. This is the way that plants uncannily solved the problem of fertilization, attesting to a high order of intelligence in plant life (which is perceived by few).

Humans do not collect nectar. Even if they did, it would be a very poor food though it sustains bees and insects well. Fertilization in this manner is necessary to certain forms of plant life to insure that seeds be created with which to propagate the species. As we know, plant life is stationary. Once it has created its seed progeny, a new problem arises, that of scattering the seeds so they will flourish. How did this uncanny wisdom in nature accomplish this?

Among the many solutions was that of creating yet another food around the seed or seeds. In attracting consumption of this food by mobile creature, there was the incidental distribution of its seeds to areas where they would not compete for space and raw materials with the parent plant. Of course, that same immense wisdom dic-

64

tated the creation of seeds that were unappetizing so they would be discarded rather than consumed.

But the greatest wisdom of all, perhaps, was that which created the food package to proportionately meet the precise needs of its eaters: Those creatures which, in taking and becoming dependent on these foods, became the fruit plant's biological symbiont. That this method of seed distribution was successful is evidenced by the thousands of kinds of fruits created around seeds in nature. Fruits attract human senses in nature and are gourmet delights in their natural ripened state, which ensures their survival. Also, fruits contain no poisons in the fresh ripened state whereas almost all plants and seeds contain components which we cannot metabolize, hence are toxic directly or indirectly.

Fruits in nature are in a predigested form when they ripen. Fruits ripen when their seeds are at a mature stage ready for reproduction. When fruits ripen, they change to brilliant colors and emit seductive fragrances to attract consumption from a biological symbiont. The tree, stalk or vine is rewarded in that its seeds are distributed, thus perpetuating its kind. They are beautiful to behold and emit captivating aromas and fragrances. This makes them irresistibly attractive to their biological symbionts. If all the water and fiber are removed from most of these fruits, the predigested carbohydrates are almost all the same, about 350 calories per 100 grams on average, more than enough to meet the energy needs of biological symbionts. This is about 88% of solids.

In like manner fruits supply from 4 to 8 grams of amino acids per 100 grams, almost every one of them with all the essential amino acids in about the proportions that humans require, plus, of course, other amino acids. The average amino acid content is about the same as mother's milk for a growing baby. The average is about 6% of solids. When sufficient calories have been consumed to meet caloric needs, intake is almost double our actual daily amino acid shortfall from recycling.

Further, the fatty acids from almost all fruits other than avocados and olives constitute about 1% to 5% of solids other than fiber. These fatty acids are liberal in their supply of the essential fatty acids. The average fatty acid content of fruits is about 2%.

But, importantly, fruits are rich in mineral matter in the most utilizable form in all nature! Of its solids about 3% are minerals including, of course, ample calcium to meet our needs if we do not eat more than 20% acid-forming foods and if we do not cook and derange fruit nutrients.

Of the labeled macronutrients there are vitamins which are really micronutrients, so little as not to be ordinarily measurable. A year of the RDAs for vitamins would not fill a sewing thimble! Yet fruits supply many multiples of the RDAs of vitamins in almost every instance. For instance, vitamin C in fruits sufficient to meet our caloric needs is about ten times as much, on average, as the RDA for it.

As humans developed exclusively on fruits, they failed to develop water drinking faculties. Those on the fruit diet have 60% to 70% less need for water than those on the conventional diet, primarily because pathogens require inordinate amounts of water to hold them in suspension and carry them out of the body. Fruits supply ample water in its purest form to meet our needs. Fruitarians do not normally drink water but make as many trips to the urinal as anyone.

As a last consideration, fruits are alkaline in their metabolic end products. The body readily excretes excess alkalis whereas it must neutralize objectionable acids and excrete them if able. (Arthritis, bursitis, rheumatism, gout and yet other problems are caused by the body's inability to excrete base salts from acid neutralization, usually calcium salts. For instance the uric acid of meats are neutralized into calcium urate crystals because we do not secrete the enzyme, uricase, as carnivores do. These salts have an affinity for cartilage in joints. Also having this affinity are the acid end products of grains, oxalic acids in vegetables like spinach, chard, beets and lamb's quarter, most cooked foods, and meats.)

We are biological symbionts of fruit-bearing plants and in nature would eat very little besides fruits. Despite all this, there's no particular harm in eating green leafy vegetables, stalks, stems and their fresh juices in the raw state. Even some steaming or conservative cooking of tubers, stalks, stems, roots, corns and selected legumes and grains (preferably sprouted), are not sufficiently deleterious to seriously harm our health. Of course, there are some toxic results from eating all this cooked fare and we're better off without them. Yet, I repeat, there is no great harm in their consumption relative to what is suffered from conventional fare.

When ripened, fruits convert their carbohydrate components into glucose and fructose, simple sugars we can use without further digestion. Their enzymes convert their proteins into amino acids and their fats into fatty acids and glycerols. Thus, when we eat fruits, all we need do is savor their goodness. The fruit portions, that is, mesocarps, were specifically compounded to attract biological symbionts. Fruits perfectly meet their nutrient needs with predigested nutrients. For humans, no other food compares with fruits in satisfying all needs including, of course, our requirement for delicious soul-exalting fare.

Are we a species of fruit-eaters? I'm sure that you will agree through your own senses that fruits would be your primary food in a state of nature. Would you, in nature, relish ripe grapes, peaches, melons, bananas, apples, plums, oranges, mangoes, avocados, tomatoes, figs, berries and the thousands of other fruits? Would fruits attract your eye, tantalize your sense of smell, and be a gustatory delight in their raw natural ripe state? Would you prefer anything that occurs in nature to a juicy sweet watermelon? Man has always had a love affair going with fruits. Even through all his perversions, he has continued to relish fruits.

Fruits are the natural food of humans and the only food category ideally suited to all their faculties. This does not mean we should eat fruits totally and exclusively in our present circumstances, but it does mean that, in nature, that's all we ate as attested to by anthropological evidence scientists have uncovered, notably Dr. Alan Walker of Johns Hopkins University.

Fruits really have it all; all that it took to make us into superb human beings; all that is required to sustain us in a healthy state insofar as food contributes to this condition; and all that we need to live a long, rewarding and happy life.

* * *

Conclusions and Observations

That we are biologically fruitarians is an inescapable conclusion on every count that we can relevantly and validly cite. What does this mean in practical application? Almost everyone you meet will condemn fruitarian fare. Almost everyone thinks from the standpoint that sickness is inevitable and must be prevented whereas, in fact, diseases simply will not occur unless we cause them, either through deficiencies or intoxications or both. If you eat 70% to 80% fruits and the balance in leafy green salads along with conservatively cooked tubers, roots and even grain products along with some raw nuts and seeds, you will not significantly or even noticeably impair yourself assuming, of course, that your other practices are good.

There are social considerations that make some concessions on dietary intake preferable to social ostracism. In my own case I merely tell those who inquire about why I'm not eating, or who urge me to eat meat dishes or obnoxious fare, that I'm on a special diet and that, while I'd love to have what is being offered, I don't dare touch it lest I suffer problems. You'll inevitably be assailed by those who tell you about vitamin B-12 deficiency and anemia. This vitamin is created by both fermentative and putrefactive bacteria. Grass contains no vitamin B-12 either, yet we are bade to eat beef liver among others for B-12. Mother Nature was, indeed, provident and provides us amply with our B-12 needs from our intestinal tract through symbiotic bacterial flora just as with other animals in nature. Experiments with baboons on a fruit diet only for many years could not induce a B-12 deficiency in any of them.

It is also rewarding to learn that, in a research to put the fruit-eating fad to rest, Professor Meyer of the University of Pretoria fed 50 controls fruits and nuts only for a period of six months. Instead of deficiencies and disease, the controls became rather sickness-free and greatly improved in health and weight. The results were published in the February 20, 1971 issue of the *South African Medical Journal.*

* * *

Questions and Answers

Q. I know that you've said that fruits are adequate in protein, having on average as much as a mother's milk. But I have heard that if we eat extra protein as in nuts, seeds and vegetables, we'll do a lot better. Is this true?

A. I cannot definitely answer you. I can point out that the experiments in South Africa incorporated nuts into the regimen with apparent benefit. Vegetables have about four times the protein as fruits but, eaten raw with the proteins intact, it's a case of how much you can derive from cellulose encased nutrients. If you steam them conservatively, it's a question of how much the proteins are deranged while being conservatively cooked. On the other side of the ledger, it's a question if steaming, which bursts most of the cellulose membranes, makes yet more proteins available in a utile condition.

Nuts and seeds are both storage forms of protein and fats. When you get the one, you get the other. We see great praise for pumpkin, sesame, flax and sunflower seeds. We see great praise for almonds and walnuts and, on occasion, hazel nuts. Raw fats, though they take a very long time to digest, evidently give us few if any problems.

My own experience with myself and hundreds of those who write in is inconclusive. Most who write to me bespeak an inability to handle nuts. Some speak of adverse results. Some can tolerate seeds but not nuts. Personally I love nuts and seeds and can handle both very well. I especially like pecans and pine nuts, often called pignolias. Mixing the two in a nut butter (putting them through a masticating juicer such as a Champion) of about 50% each along with a little soaked sea vegetables (I relish alaris and dulse but can't stand the fishy tastes of the others) creates an excellent dressing base, vegetable dip, etc. To liquefy this somewhat I often add tomato to the mixture in the making. Go ahead and eat vegetables, seeds and nuts if they agree with you. There's no particular harm in them that I know of. Peace of mind is far more important than uncertainty.

Q. I'm a nursing mother. A fellow who knows of my primarily fruit based diet says: "B-12 is needed by the body. Your diet doesn't have any. Your body cannot manufacture it. You cannot get it from non-meat sources." I've been on this diet for a number of years and I don't buy his line. What reply can I give this guy?

A. Your acquaintance has been misled by meat industry spokespeople, vitamin peddlers, dietitians" and "nutritionists". First, the question might be asked: Where do vegetarian animals get this vitamin B-12? They don't manufacture any, either! And certainly grasses and the fare of vegetarian animals contains no vitamin B-12! Vitamin B-12 is so abundantly produced in our bodies that it is hard not to get enough! We meet our needs amply for this vitamin from bacterial by-products generated by bacterial flora from the mouth all the way down to and through the absorbing colon. According to *Guyton's Textbook of Medical Physiology*, bacteria in the upper half of the colon, called the caecum or absorbing colon, create ample vitamin B-12, vitamin K, thiamine and riboflavin. Some energy is surrendered to the body by these same bacteria in breaking down cellulose to a small extent and converting it to glucose. One milligram of B-12 will last us over two years, and healthy individuals usually carry around a five-year supply. Our needs are so minute, they are measured in picograms (billionths of a gram) and micrograms (millionths of a gram).

The fact that vegetarians and fruitarians carry less B-12 in their bloodstreams than meat eaters does not prove that we have inadequate amounts of B-12. We do not store this vitamin in our bloodstream but in the liver and other organs. We carry in our bloodstream only that which has been picked up from the colon (by intrinsic factor) and is earmarked for reserves, or which has been released from organs to meet our current needs. Meat eaters do carry more B-12 in their bloodstreams. They probably need more too, in light of their handicap in partaking of a pathogenic diet. Also, because of the double source of B-12 from meats, putrefactive products and intestinal ferments and putrefaction, their bloodstreams are contaminated. Live in full confidence that Mother nature had things right for us to start with.

Q. How can you live on fruits only? You'd have to be eating all the time. What if you tried to live on oranges only?

A. The Florida citrus industry did just that back in the 1930s. A man lived on oranges only for six years! At the end of the demonstration, the man was proclaimed to be in robust health.

To get the some 2,250 calories an average sized man needs, about 10 pounds of orange flesh daily would have to be consumed, about three pounds more than the average American takes in gross weight of conventional fare. There would be surfeits of water in the winter and quite enough during the hot summer. This is about 20 average oranges. That amount of calories would yield, in addition to caloric sufficiency, about 2,250 milligrams of vitamin C, 1,800 milligrams of calcium, 45 grams of protein, 9 grams of fats, 18 milligrams of iron, 27 grams of minerals overall—in short, more of everything than we are said to require by the RDA excepting calories which are much too high for a raw food eater.

Q. Are dried fruits as good as fresh fruits? Should we eat them at all?

A. Dried fruits are never as good as fresh ripe fruits. Yes, we should eat dried fruits when fresh fruits available to us do not meet our caloric needs. Dried fruits have lost a substantial portion of their vitamins and some of their minerals due to oxidation. Dried fruits are good primarily for their fuel value and because they do not have the disadvantages of cooked foods. They are usually ultra-sweet, thus serving as wonderful desserts when eaten with other fruits. The Hunzas live on dried fruits and some grains for months at a time during the winter/spring season. Should you eat dried fruits alone, I suggest that you rinse or clean your teeth thoroughly. Dried fruits are said to be as bad for the teeth as white sugar.

Q. Is sea salt healthful?

A. *by David Klein.* The major component of sea salt is sodium chloride. Sea salt is touted as being healthier that table salt because the former has more trace minerals and the latter is heat processed. Nonetheless, mineral salts in inorganic form are extremely toxic— they impair all of our metabolic and cellular functions. Because it is toxic, the body retains water to dilute the toxicity so we don't die. This is edema, and it can result in headaches and heart irregularity. When we are retaining water, the fluid balance in the body is out of balance and cellular transport is impaired. The body needs to maintain the fluid pressure inside the cells at a specific ratio to the fluid pressure outside of the cells. When we have extra high fluid pressure outside of the cells as a result of salt eating, the cells are not able to efficiently transport normal metabolic wastes out of the cells, thus we become more and more toxic, leading to chronic fatigue and illness.

Furthermore, the body needs to maintain specific concentration ratios of sodium to potassium inside and outside of the cells for proper functioning. A high salt diet leads to excess sodium becoming "locked into" to cells, creating cellular dysfunction. This has been linked to many modern diseases, including cancer, diabetes, hardening of arteries, hypertension, kidney disease, nervous disorders, and osteoporosis.

As long as we have salt in our diet, we cannot effectively detoxify, lose excess weight and completely heal. Once we discontinue salt, it can take many as a few years to offload all of the excess sodium. The U.S. dietary guideline makers who allow a few grams of salt in the diet every day are unaware of the toxic effects of such, or are

OK with toxic fare in the diet in moderation. Of course, a toxin is a toxin and has enervating and potentially harmful synergistic effects in any amount.

Q. Are soybeans a healthful food?

A. *by David Klein.* Soybeans and inclusive products are a poor food choice for humans. Eaten raw, straight from the plant, sprouted, or cooked without additives or flavorings, soybeans are bland and thus we would not naturally eat them. Soybean's potential nutritional value is greatly diminished by cooking—much of the proteins, vitamins and antioxidants are damaged and rendered unusable in the body. Soybeans are high in protein and starch, a combination that is difficult to digest. Furthermore, soybeans contain oligosaccharides, small short-chain sugars which we cannot digest due to our inability to secrete the appropriate enzymes. The inevitable result of eating legumes, such as soybeans, is bacterial decomposition in the gut accompanied by gas and acid waste poisoning.

Soybeans and soybean products are highly acid-forming; we need to eat a mostly alkalizing diet of fruits and vegetables to maintain health. A diet of mostly acid-forming foods acidifies the blood, leading to osteoporosis, as calcium is leached from the bones in order to neutralize the acids. Bland-tasting tofu, like most soybean products, often has toxic irritating flavorings/condiments added to render it palatable. These additives tend to impair digestion. Lastly, almost all soybeans are now genetically modified, with proven detrimental health effects.

If we want pure and naturally delicious hearty protein foods with all of the amino acids we need, nuts, seeds (raw or germinated, whole, or blended with water to make a "milk"), vegetables, avocado and young soft coconuts are superior, and the most healthful choices.

* * *

Research Yields a Bombshell of a Surprise!
Scientist Uncovers Paradise Diet
as Natural to Humans

The prestigious *New York Times* newspaper, in its May 15, 1979 issue, surprised your author more by printing an article than the surprise they express by the findings revealed. The gist of this article concerns work done by an anthropologist, Dr. Alan Walker of Johns Hopkins University in Maryland. Dr. Walker has come to the startling conclusion that early humans were fruit eaters—eaters of nothing but fruit. This comes as quite a bombshell from a noted publication that has a vested interest in a heavy meat-eating society.

By careful examination of fossil teeth and fossilized remains of humans with the aid of electron microscopes and other sophisticated tools, Dr. Walker and other researchers are absolutely certain that our ancestors, up to a point in relatively recent history, were fruitarians. A cursory study of biology will reveal that we are indeed frugivores, even if written by meat-eating professors, which most of our biologists are.

* * *

Addressing the Charges

Addressing the charge that fruits are protein poor and are inadequate in essential amino acids

The charge is made that fruits are protein poor and possessed of insufficient amino acids to sustain us. It is true that, if you compare a banana in the dry state with its 5% amino acid (protein) content to a soybean in the dry state with a 34% protein content, the banana is, indeed, protein poor. But the nutrient content of any food has relevance only to our need for it. So we must understand our need for amino acids (if we eat proteins, they must be

74

broken down into amino acids before absorption) relative to our needs.

If you try to eat the protein of soy beans raw, you can't manage it—you aren't able to digest them. If you cook soy bean protein, the amino acids are substantially or totally deaminated, thus giving you cooked carbohydrates and lots of putrefiable nitrogenous materials. Putrefaction of these materials begets indole, skatole, mercaptans, cadaverine, neurine, putrescine, muscarine, ammonia, methane gas, ptomatropine, leukomaines and ptomaines, hydrogen sulfide, carbon dioxide and yet other poisons. If absorbed from the ileum and caecum, and many are, they give rise to the intoxication that leads to ailments, sicknesses or diseases.

Of course, we don't get proteins from fruits as proteins. When ripe, fruits are in a predigested state. The carbohydrates are delivered to the consumers of fruits as fructose and glucose. The protein complement is yielded as ready-to-absorb amino acids. And fruits deliver fats as simple fatty acids—monoglycerides/glycerol.

As to the charge that fruits have no protein or inadequate protein, we need point only to the fallacy devised by the meat and dairy trusts to ensnare their unwitting servants called nutritionists and dietitians. Of course, the deluding of the population at large is standard practice as well. But this propaganda is shot full of holes as a few facts and logical reasoning therefrom will readily reveal.

A growing human baby gets a mono diet of its mother's milk for many months, even a year, before it touches any other food. At least that's the way it is in nature and with hygienic mothers. Mother's milk for her rapidly developing infant contains all its nutrient needs. But, alas, her milk contains 1.1% protein! Or 7% protein dry weight, less than is contained by oranges, watermelons, paw paws and many other fruits.

Surely no one can, with sanity, argue that a grown-up can require more protein (amino acids) than a growing child relative to its weight or as a percentage of its diet. If anything, the grown-up who has attained full development requires less protein than a nursing tot. Demonstrably, adults can get adequate protein on less than half a percent of dietary intake!

The RDA for protein is said to be 56 grams daily for an average man of 70 kilograms or 154 pounds. This figure is well over twice that established by tests by Dr. Chittenden of Yale, Dr. Mark Hegsted of Harvard, or Dr. Hinhede in Denmark and many others of late. Further, there are groups of robust people in the Caribbean who thrive on an average intake of 10 to 15 grams of protein daily. (They eat cassava or manioc as a primary, almost total item of diet.) Keeping in mind that the body obtains over 90% of its protein needs by recycling its proteinaceous wastes, it becomes somewhat evident that protein needs in humans have been grossly exaggerated. The meat, dairy, poultry and fish industries have made their mark, even on those who reject animal products as foods.

Dr. Hegsted and others have established the protein need (amino acid need) of 150 pound males as 21 grams. The RDA is arrived at by adding 33% as a margin of safety and then doubling that to accommodate those whose protein metabolism is poor.

That we are natural fruit eaters is proven beyond refutation by our own natural disposition as well as the scientific data available. Fruits must have (and will continue to have as will be demonstrated) furnished our nutrient needs adequately including our amino acid needs. For instance, our need of vitamin C and some other vitamins must be furnished wholly by our foods. There's no way the body can synthesize them. Why? We're told that these vitamins are so abundant in the natural human dietary that humans long since lost the faculties to create them. The body's faculties for creating needs are lost if these needs are amply and reliably furnished from the outside. That principle applies across the spectrum of nutrient needs! Why are we dependent on essential amino acids? For one very compelling reason: Our natural diet furnishes us adequately and reliably with the amino acids we require but cannot synthesize.

Then we must face charges that we need so much of this or that essential amino acid on a daily basis, yet another RDA, so to speak. And that fruits are woefully short of them. Much of our exaggerated RDAs are derived by the doubling practice of the NRC of the National Academy of Sciences. We know that the human body of the average man synthesizes about 230 grams of protein daily! We also know that over 90% of this protein generation is supplied by recycling protein losses of the system. Of all the amino acids involved, no studies exist showing how much of their need is supplied by recycling. Might we not logically assume that 90% of our exaggerated RDA is likewise supplied by recycling?

Again, our natural diet necessarily had to adequately furnish our essential amino acid needs, otherwise we would not have lost our faculties for creating them—providing that we did at one time create them or that our dietary was never less than adequate in them.

Can we continue to say that fruits are protein poor? Or deficient in essential amino acids? In view that if protein in fruits constitute one percent of our diet, as much as required by a rapidly growing infant, we must conclude that fruits are protein (really amino acid) adequate. When a very active 154 pound man takes in some 2,250 calories of fruits, the protein complement of 160 calories (40 grams) is nearly twice as much as actually required. And, as most fruits do contain all the essential amino acids, I would adjudge that fruits amply supply human needs for each and every amino acid.

Methinks that most of the charges and posturing amounts to tilting at ghostly windmills, ghosts created by our agricultural department which is very subservient to the meat, milk and egg industries as well as the trusts certain controlling interests have built around these animal products. They often impose their misinformation or disinformation upon us as valid findings. Too many of us are victims of this sort of thinking. It's surprising we ever got this far as fruitarians when....

History bears out beyond refutation that humans have been fruit eaters during their sojourn on earth, excepting a period beginning during the ice ages. Even then, a preponderance of our ancestors still ate and subsisted on fruits. Most migrated south to warmer climates and continued to eat fruits. Grain eating is not more than 10,000 years old and hardly registers on the scale of time relative to human existence. Meat eating, though much older than that, was mostly confined to northerly peoples. Almost all mythology is built around trees and fruits, around climatic factors and the sun which affected trees. Only relatively recent mythologies and legends connect humans to grain culture and animal husbandry.

Addressing the charge that fruits are deficient in calcium and fruitarian children have stunted growth and are abnormally small

To explore this charge I made charts of a number of fruits and their compositions. Our fuel needs can be amply met by fruits. Calcium, as well as the other spectrum of nutrients, are components of every gram of fruit. When we have eaten sufficient fruit to supply our caloric needs, say about 2,250 calories for a very active 154 pounder, how much of our RDA for calcium have we met? The RDA is set at 800 milligrams per day. Of course, we know that this RDA is three or four times too high, for Bantu women in Africa get along very well on 300 to 400 mg. of calcium per day and suffer no osteoporosis while their American counterparts may take in 1,000 mg. and still suffer osteoporosis!

This is so because so much of the calcium intake of Americans are inorganic as in supplements and deranged to an inorganic state as in cooked foods. Further, the average American eats so many acid-forming foods like meats and grains as to bind, even rob us of much of our calcium intake. Further, the vaunted calcium in milk is mostly unavailable to us because we do not secrete rennin to break down the casein and milk has so much phosphorus as to bind it anyway. And there are really free acids as in vinegars, fermented milks, rotted cheeses, uric acids of meats, phosphoric acids of soft drinks, etc., which also bind lots of calcium and alkaline minerals.

Oranges, a widely consumed fruit, when eaten sufficiently to meet caloric needs or about 2,250 calories for a very active 154 pound man, have about 2,050 milligrams of calcium, 2 1/2 times the RDA. Apples have 315 milligrams, apricots 782, cantaloupes

1,078, figs 1,130 and bananas, upon which whole populations subsist, 224. Be it noted that banana eating societies have excellent bone formation by all standards. Grapes have 440 mg. of calcium, dates 530, mangos 370, pineapples 785, watermelon 640 and so on down the line. Obviously, fruits supply us amply with our calcium needs. And the saying that fruit eaters suffer stunted growth does not withstand serious inquiry. Statuesque Greeks were fruit eaters.

While it is true that fruit eaters are smaller than their meat-eating, milk-drinking, poison-ingesting counterparts, we must recognize in them the disease called giantism. Our average height today is eight inches more than it was in such ancestors as George Washington, Benjamin Franklin, Thomas Jefferson, etc. Even seven footers, rather common today, were quite rare a mere 50 years ago.

Addressing the charge that fruits do not have any vitamin B-12

Fruits are charged as having no vitamin B-12. Guilty! The same can be said of almost all vegetarian fare, even herbage that animals eat. Only meats, fermented and putrefied foods such as cheese and certain kinds of algae have what is termed sufficient vitamin B-12 to meet our needs. But if animal fare such as grasses, leaves, grains, herbs and fruits do not furnish us or animals with vitamin B-12, how do their organs come to be so rich in it? How come the organs of fruit-eating primates are rich in it? How is it that fruitarian societies are not anemic from lack of vitamin B-12?

The truth is that humans, like all other animals, obtain ample supplies of vitamin B-12 from bacterial production in their intestines from cobalamin, provided the mineral cobalt is in the context of foods. Even garlic eaters usually do not destroy enough of their symbiotic intestinal flora to deny themselves an adequate supply of vitamin B-12. If you number the anemics, you'll find most are meat eaters! Further, almost all have lost the ability to secrete intrinsic factor, the transport medium for vitamin B-12. I adjudge the charge that fruit eaters are anemic to be without any substantive evidence whatsoever. Remember, it's the meat, dairy and other trusts that originate such propaganda, oops, sorry, disinformation.

Addressing the charge that fruitarians suffer nutritional imbalances and deficiencies

The charge that fruit eaters will suffer nutritional imbalances and deficiencies likewise finds no basis. Fruits are the only foods that create a food package to proportionately meet the nutrient needs of their biological symbionts, though many animals have adapted to many foods other than fruits. In fact, fruits, eaten according to their season, furnish us with every nutrient factor, known and unknown, in plenteousness greater than we require. Again, the ancient Greeks whom we admire so much for their statuesque bodies, were fruit eaters. Most ate heavily of apples, dates, oranges, olives, figs and grapes. Many of the Greek and Roman gods are ascriptions born of reverence for fruit trees and food-bearing plants, notably Apollo which literally means apple.

Addressing the charge that fruit eaters cannot maintain weight and become too thin

The charge that fruit eaters are too thin is not borne out by even the merest inquiry. Personally, I did lose from 200 pounds to 126 on a mostly fruit diet. But on the same diet and regimen I gained back to the 150 pound range. I had excellent muscular development on a diet consisting almost entirely of fruits with very few nuts and seeds.

As before pointed out, the Greeks thrived on fruitarian diets. Pythagoras, one of the giants of Grecian literature, philosophy and mathematics, was a fruitarian and had a whole school of followers who, likewise, became fruitarians. Actually, the teachings of Pythagoras very much parallel the teachings of Gautama Buddha with whose teachings Pythagoras became conversant on his sojourn in India. Buddha was, in essence, a tree worshipper as were fruitarian societies. Buddha's love affair with bananas is well-known. In India bananas are known as the food of the wise. Bacchus, the god of wine, is portrayed as heavily overweight and this was attributed to

80

fig gluttony. I maintain my weight very well on a mostly fruitarian diet with some nuts, seeds and vegetables. So do others.

Addressing the charge that fruit eaters become over-alkaline and often suffer alkalosis

The charge that fruit eaters are over-alkaline and often suffer alkalosis is, likewise, baseless. We humans can harmlessly excrete excess alkaline end-products, but, if we get excess acid-forming end-products as from meats, animal products, cereal foods, breads, etc., we really have problems! The body must rob its bones and other alkaline stores and structures for the alkalis, mostly calcium, necessary to neutralize the acid end-products.

Whoever originated this charge of "alkalosis" simply did not know or ignored physiology. I have had alkalosis but not in the 24 years I've been mostly fruitarian. When I was a conventional eater I had acidosis (heartburn) so much I would take too many antacid tablets or too much bicarbonate of soda and get the same discomfort, but from alkalosis.

Everyone is fruitarian by nature. Our development in nature was fruitarian. To say that we require an alkaline end-product diet on the one hand and then say that we cannot handle alkalis is contradictory. If nature is anything at all, it is certainly provident. Eating up to 20% acid-forming products presents no great problem. Fruits and vegetables are, for practical purposes, alkaline in metabolic end-products. Most nuts and grains are acid-forming. Legumes are acid-forming unless sprouted or eaten in the fresh green state. Conventionally cooked foods, even if of normally alkaline-forming vegetables, become acid-forming. Conservatively cooked alkaline-forming foods remain alkaline in end-products. All animal products are acid-forming, including milk, except blood which is alkaline and butter which is neutral.

Addressing the charge that fruits have too much sugar

Obviously this charge is made by those who have not weighed or cogitated upon the considerations. Or those who refuse to recognize the evidence. First, about 90% of our nutrient requirements aside from water are for monosaccharides (simple sugars are glucose, fructose, glycerose and galactose) for energy. Until you've met this need, it is ridiculous to cry "too much sugar." Sugar in fruits comes to us predigested, hence it can't be beyond our digestive capacity, though it may go on down the intestinal tube if ingested beyond absorptive capacity which, too, is unlikely because of the satiety factor which limits fruit-eating to actual replenishment needs.

Fruit sugars are said to be absorbed "too fast," but they do not present nearly the problem with their fructose content as digested starches which are all glucose. Recent research has proven that the glucose (rated at 100 as a sugar load factor) of starches (mostly grains and tubers in our case) is absorbed just as fast as fruit sugars. Moreover, they "storm" the body's sugar metabolizing faculties more greatly than do fruit sugars, with the component fructose (rated at 29 as a sugar load factor). If we eat "too much sugar," that is, caloric values exceeding our needs, then obviously we've overeaten. In the case of sugar, the surplus is either stored as fats or harmlessly excreted.

Lets look at starches, often called complex carbohydrates. These must be heated to be broken down from long chain polysaccharides or starch. Heating dextrinizes starches. However, because there are no immediate sugars to absorb for appestat control, overeating of dextrinized starches is endemic. And many athletes intentionally eat heavily of starchy foods (dextrinized by heat) as in "carbohydrate loading." As dextrinized starches are converted to glucose, once absorption starts, according to recent research, our bloodstream is hit with as big a sugar load as fruits present!

As to excess sugar, we're more likely to get it from starches on which we're more likely to overeat than from fruits which quickly satisfy the appestat. In the case of heated starches, unless heated at very low temperatures for an extended period of time, our fungal and bacterial flora can readily ferment it, thus intoxicating us to some extent. Uncooked sugars are not fermentable until they have been oxidized, a process unlikely to happen with these quickly absorbed foods unless other factors delay their absorption. When explored and examined, the charge of "excessive sugar" vanishes.

Addressing the charge that fruits,
especially dried fruits, ruin the teeth

It is commonly believed that our "sweet tooth" was installed by nature only to get us into trouble. "Yield not unto temptation" lest your teeth be ruined, is a modern day dental admonition. To give this charge credence we must necessarily regard Dr. Alan Walker, the noted Johns Hopkins University anthropologist, as mistaken. Some are quick to reason that our forebears did not eat fruits exclusively, as he says for, had they, they couldn't possibly have had any teeth left to become fossilized. And, equally so, it was devilish of God to make us fruitarians, place us in an orchard called the Garden of Eden, and command us to eat only fruits (Gen. 1: 29-30) and then leave us wide open to tooth decay by those very foods.

Dentists have long had cautions about sugar eating because it causes tooth decay. Most will not admit that teeth are mostly sabotaged from the inside rather than the outside. But let us look at the nonsugar eating Eskimos who did and still do, for the most part, eat only fats and proteins. Their intake is about 200 grams of fat daily and about an equal amount of protein, all in the raw state as they do not cook. Yet the average Eskimo has lost all of his or her teeth by the age of 30! This is self-evidence that a heavy acid-forming diet sabotages tooth integrity. Of course it does likewise with their bones, for they have widespread osteoporosis. In their far north habitat a 40-year-old is into old age!

I have asked dentists about this and they categorically deny that the body will rob calcium and other base minerals from teeth though they readily admit that the body will rob alkaline minerals from bones to maintain chemical homeostasis. I have also asked about the claim that sugars cause tooth decay as it involves fruit sugars, especially of dried fruit. I'm still waiting for substantive proof that they do.

Addressing the charge that excess sugars turn to tryclycerides and cause overweight

This is some charge to make against fruitarians who are in no ways fat! There's a whole country of fruit-eaters in the jungles of Nicaragua called the Mesquito Indians. Are there any fatties or giants among them? From pictures I've seen, there's nary a one. The same goes for chimpanzees who habitually overeat on fruit when available (as much as 40 bananas per creature according to Jane Goodall). Personally, I was grossly overweight until I undertook the fruitarian diet. Now I'm normal in weight and have been for the more than 24 years that I've been primarily a fruitarian.

Fatness is a feast or famine response of the body to distress which threatens the body. This survival mechanism causes abnormal weight gain in anticipation of possible famine. As fruits never intoxicate and distress the body as conventional fare does, this response does not, in fact, occur on a fruit diet. I've seen obese persons undertake a fruitarian diet and eat double what they should, yet lose weight reliably! Fats are gained on conventional diets and lost on fruit diets! This is a charge that exactly reverses the truth.

Addressing the charge that today's fruits are developed by plant breeders to be too sweet and are nutritionally inferior by comparison with fruits in their ancient natural setting

I know this charge to be without relevant substantiveness on two counts:

1. Those making the statements do not have composition data about fruits of yore even though there are still lots of wild fruits to be had, and....

2. Composition data about today's fruits reflect them to be nutritionally adequate even if they are not as nutritious as their forerunners were in nature.

Yes, fruits are continually being hybridized and bred as new strains and varieties. And while flavor and sweetness are striven for in the development of new varieties and strains, nutritionally they are about the same—some are indeed inferior to the natural counterpart but some are more nutritious also! Further, with today's knowledge of growing super nutritious fruits with mineralization techniques, especially trace minerals from the sea often given as foliar sprays, there is no reason that today's fruits can't be equal to or superior to the natural product of yesteryear.

* * *

What Does a Fruitarian Eat?

Anyone who eats a predominantly fruit diet is a fruitarian! Anyone who eats more than 50% of his diet as fruit solids (considering all foods eaten on the basis of solids only) is a fruitarian.

I am the 154 pound man, plus or minus, who just happens to be the dietary 70 kilograms around which dietary requirements are formulated in most analyses. I am very active physically and mentally. I maintain my weight by weight-lifting and exertive exercises for a net time of only 10 minutes weekly. I am 5'6". My aerobic exercises aggregate a net of about 35 minutes weekly, much of it as short sprints and jumping jacks. I run only about three miles weekly and sprint perhaps 1,500 yards total. Both jumping jacks and sprints are energizers like you wouldn't believe unless you've experienced their lifts. As a mostly mental worker, I have Baroque, Classical and Renaissance music as background. This facilitates thinking as well as learning. But nothing awakens me and makes me more alert than a 100 yard sprint, a mile run or 60 to 70 jumping jacks. My crossword puzzling and chess playing ability is quickly and immensely enhanced. As I do lots of writing, a burst of activity as in sprinting does wonders for energizing and sharpening my thinking powers. I've analyzed a week of my diet by solid weight of the respective foods I've eaten. The foods were as follows in a very cool spring week in Michigan. Temperatures were in the 30s to 50s for the most part.

Food	Wt. as eaten	Wt. as solids	Calories
Grapes	4 lbs.	12 oz.	1,080
Muskmelon	6 lbs.	8 oz.	810
Bananas	6 lbs.	24 oz.	2,310
Oranges w/o peel	8 lbs.	18 oz.	1,780
Lemon Juice	4 oz.	4 oz.	30
Papaya	1 lb.	2 oz.	195
Dates, dried	1 lb.	12 oz.	1,235
Raisins	15 oz.	12.5 oz.	1,260
Apples	3 lbs.	9 oz.	740
Avocados	20 oz.	6 oz.	1,020
Strawberries	1 lb.	2 oz.	170
Pears	11 oz.	2 oz.	185
Squash Seeds	2.5 oz.	2.4 oz.	420
Sunflower Seeds	2.5 oz.	2.4 oz.	460
Almonds	3 oz.	2.8 oz.	510
Pecans	6 oz.	5.8 oz.	1,275
Sweet Red Peppers	2 lbs.	3 oz.	300
Tomatoes	5 lbs.	6 oz.	495
Lettuce, Bibb	22 oz.	1.1 oz.	80
Bok Choy	28 oz.	1.4 oz.	105
Dulse	.1 oz.	.1 oz.	5
TOTAL INTAKE	44 lbs., 2 oz.	8 lbs., 2 oz.	14,285

As you see, your author is a fair eater! I eat on an average of six occasions daily, holding that little and often is better than three belly-boggling meals per day. My single largest meal is always a salad with nuts or avocados in the evening. My salads are mostly fruits, consisting of tomatoes, red peppers and avocados. I usually add bok choy or lettuce with a sprinkling of dulse powder. I eat well over 99% of my intake in the raw condition. On rare occasions I might have a baked potato when eating out with others if the potato is baked "rare."

Note that the diet averages 2,000 calories daily. You need more calories when running and living in the North. You require more just to maintain body heat. In the summer my foods have a much higher water content and my caloric intake is only about 1,600 per day. Note that of a total solid intake of eight pounds, less than one pound of nonfruits were taken, almost all being nuts and seeds which I ate rather heavily of all winter and will eat very little of during the summer. Note that the total vegetable intake (lettuce, bok choy and dulse) amounted to only 2.6 ounces of solids out of 130 total ounces of intake, about 2% of the diet. Green leafy vegetables yield folic acid, an essential B complex vitamin. Believe me, half a pound of lettuce and/or bok choy a day is quite a bit of vegetable eating.

While tomatoes and red peppers are considered vegetables, they are really fruits. Note that dulse was taken. It was in a powdered form and was added to salads consisting of tomatoes, bok choy or lettuce, peppers and either nuts, seeds or avocados with lemon juice. Dulse gives you usable trace minerals which are rather sparse in land grown foods—it's a kind of nutrient insurance.

Among my many phone calls are often questions like: "But, Mr. Fry, why don't you eat fresh raw sprouts? They're especially healthful. And you can eat fresh green peas and corn raw. Why don't you do so?" Well, I've never eaten any sprouts yet that I liked except for sunflower sprouts. On the other hand, please tell me, what are the unique nutrients or qualities in sprouts? Highly vaunted alfalfa sprouts, which are a current craze, contain a substance, canavanine, which we, unlike horses and other animals, secrete no enzyme to break down. Canavanine is a carcinogen.

As to fresh green peas and corn still in the sugar stage, I do like them. As a farm boy I raided the garden and fields for these and other fruits and vegetables. But now, if I eat them, I get sleepier sooner and sleep longer. I experience an unaccustomed thirst. My stomach feels heavier. Moreover, my exercising is off somewhat in the morning—I bomb out on the sprints sooner. I find myself clearing my throat more. And my thinking is not as sharp. After a meal of these foods it's more difficult for me to get going. I eat what I like most for that makes me feel the best. I love eating mostly all-dessert meals.

Another question concerns my protein intake. Believe me, I have to shave off a lot of it every day. If your protein intake is too low and your reserves are low (we store up to five pounds of protein as labile proteins and mucopolysaccharides), the body will not make any proteins available for hair which is mostly of protein. While proteins are more than adequately supplied by fruits (Dr. Hegsted of Harvard University says we need only 21 grams daily—the body recycles more than 200 grams of its proteinaceous wastes), I ingest fully 50 grams daily. I also think that fruitarians have longer lived cells, hence require less protein than conventional eaters who require 21 grams daily. The Carib Indians get by nicely on 12 grams daily while eating cassava roots or manioc, known to us as tapioca.

7
A General Guide to Food Selection

One way in which to pinpoint the pathogenicity or salubriousness of foods is their metabolic endpoint character. Acid-forming foods are pathogenic unless offset with alkaline end-product foods. The diet should consist at each meal of at least 80% of alkaline reaction foods. Foods that result in alkaline end-products are:

• All raw vegetables.

• All raw fruits including high acid fruits such as lemons, limes, grapefruit, oranges, etc.

• All fresh raw green beans, peas and their sprouts.

Foods that result in acid end products are all heavy protein content foods including:

• All meats including fish.

• All animal products including milk but excepting blood and butter. (We cannot get calcium from milk because it is tied up in the casein which later becomes soil for putrefactive bacteria.)

• All legumes or bean family members in their storage form of proteins, fats and starches except lima beans. This includes peanuts, which are widely consumed. Lima beans contain a deadly poison in their storage form, as do garbanzo beans.

• All nuts and seeds excepting almonds, chestnuts and coconuts.

• All grains excepting millet.

When eating acid-forming foods in a meal, the meal must be predominantly of alkaline forming vegetables. Most fruits will not do, as they are digestively incompatible with all protein, starchy and fatty foods. See Dr. Shelton's booklet *Food Combining Made Easy* and our food combining chart.

Criteria for the selection of best foods

First criterion - *Can the food be eaten in its natural state? Is the food palatable, that is delectable or delicious? Can it be eaten with keen relish in its natural state?*

If a food cannot be eaten with joy and delight to individuals in normal health with unperverted tastes, then the food receives a very low rating or no rating value. Eating should be a gustatory delight. If a food is a taste delight it receives a perfect score and a lower score commensurate with its delectability.

If the food cannot be ingested in its natural or raw state, that is, uncooked, unprocessed and otherwise untampered with, it does not belong in the human diet and receives a rating accordingly. We humans were for millions of years adapted to a diet obtained directly from nature in its fresh raw natural state. This determines the character of our diet and also the manner in which we were accustomed to ingesting it.

Therefore, cooking and processing foods to make them palatable is unacceptable to the Natural Hygienist. Cooking destroys enzymes totally. While a healthy individual will synthesize some 1,000 enzymes required for digestion, assimilation and utilization of foods, the body is, nevertheless, dependent upon the enzymic action of the foods for the most perfect digestion. Consequently, it is absolutely essential that our foods have their full complement of enzymes intact.

Cooking is the worst practice humans have adopted. It destroys not only the enzymes but deranges and destroys almost all known food factors. Cooking disorganizes, oxidizes and makes nonusable a food's mineral content. It deaminizes the food's protein content thus rendering it worthless in human nutrition. Cooking reduces the value of a food from its wholesome state all the way down to worthless ashes, depending on the degree of cooking to which it has been subjected. To the extent that a food has been cooked—reduced to inorganic minerals, caramelized sugars and starches, co-agulated and deaminized proteins, poisonous-acrolein laden fats, devitalized vitamins and loss of fuel and other values—it is not only worthless but the ash becomes toxic debris in the body. That cooked foods are poisonous in the body is easily demonstrable. The white corpuscle count doubles and triples after eating it! So the rule is this: If we can't eat the food "raw," if it is not delicious and palatable in its natural living state it is not a food for us!

RATING: O to 25 on our scale of evaluation.

Second criterion - *Does the food introduce harmful or toxic substances into our digestive system?*

If the food is proper to the human diet it must contain NO noxious or unwelcome substances. We do not want poisons in our system, no matter how little or how "mild." Anything that interferes with vital activities or destroys cells and tissue is poisonous to our system.

RATING: 0 to minus (-) 100 on our scale of evaluation, depending on degree of toxicity.

Third criterion - *Is the food easy of digestion and assimilation?*

Foods to which we humans are ideally adapted are easy of digestion and assimilation with a minimum of vital energy being necessary for their digestion and assimilation. To be of greatest value to us foods must be efficiently digested and assimilated, granting, of course, that we have unimpaired digestive systems.

Humans have become highly efficient at digesting and assimilating foods to which they, in nature, became adapted. Millions of years of development made certain foods very easy of digestion— we developed constitutions, enzymes and processes that appropriated, digested and assimilated certain foods with a minimum expenditure of vital resources and time.

RATING: 0 to 25 on our scale of evaluation.

Fourth Criterion - *Does the food contribute a broad range of nutrients? Does the food possess great biological value for us?*

I have appraised the foods listed herein for many factors.

Though many foods are rather complete in their range of nutrients, none are suitable for a mono diet such as is for cattle. But most of the foods rated are quite suitable for mono meals. And, certainly, if properly combined, these foods furnish all the nutrients we humans need.

The problem is not that we should eat a great variety in hopes of making sure to get all the nutrients needed, but rather to eat simply to afford our bodies every opportunity to easily digest and appropriate what the foods offer. What does it matter the range of nutrients we put into our bodies if we ingest them in such manner as to vitiate and tax the digestive process such that, instead of appreciating our good intentions, we fail to derive the goodness intended and penalize our bodies and rob it of nutrients as well? We should never take more than four or five different foods at a single properly prepared and combined meal. Almost no preparation other than cleansing is necessary but we must make sure to eat in strictly compatible combinations. The ideal is a single food per meal! There is no particular penalty in eating two to four different items at a meal if they are compatible in the digestive process.

To really simplify the digestive process and to assure yourself of easy digestion on a continuing basis, we may select a rather narrow range of foods according to the season and stick with them. For instance we may make one meal a day of just bananas with some lettuce and celery and another meal of a salad and nuts. This can go on day after day in the winter season. In summer we might have melon rather consistently for just one meal and at a second meal of the day, a salad with nuts or some fresh food of a starchy or proteinaceous character. The objective is a diet to which we are biologically adapted that gives the highest potential for wonderful health.

The ratings given herein are arrived at based on data available to me and my appraisal of it and other factors. I have taken into account the contribution to nutrition a food may make in the matter of calories, vitamins, minerals, enzymic factors, hormones, proteins, auxones and other beneficent food factors. Keep in mind that most foods are fairly complete in themselves if they are seeds or nuts, though this does not necessarily mean they are complete in human nutrition.

Green leaves must be accorded the highest and most complete range of nutrients. This is one of the primary reasons we must have them often in our diet for the best health (that is, if we're eating). Of course the body is provident—missing them on occasion is not particularly harmful and would not prove disastrous unless we missed them for some length of time.

While this rating chart does not spell out the nutrient contents—that knowledge not being necessary—we should plan our meals so that we receive the benefit of foods that complement each other in their nutrient contents essential in human nutrition.

RATING: O to 50 in our scale of evaluation.

Other considerations not rated

Is the food acid-forming in metabolic reaction? Is it alkaline in metabolic reaction?

The value of a food in human nutrition is not determined by these considerations, but the human diet must be overwhelmingly of alkaline-forming foods. Generally nuts, legumes and cereals are acid-forming. Nuts are quite beneficial in the human diet, whereas humans do not have the equipment to properly digest legumes (except in sprouted or fresh green state) and cereals.

Is the food economical? Do we get good nutritive value for our money?

A food's value to us must also be gauged by its cost versus its utility. For instance we can sprout mung beans and receive some of our best nutrition for just a fraction of the cost of the same values in other foods.

Is the food generally available in its fresh natural state?

This, too, is a consideration. We must eat our foods as nature delivers them to us. We can make little use of foods that have been tampered with, ground, cut up, peeled, cooked, preserved, canned, frozen, etc. Even sun-dried foods are not nearly as wholesome as in their fresh state. Raisins, figs, dates, apricots and pears, for instance, are great foods in their fresh state with all their original water content. Dried they lose much of their vitality but, on the other hand, they are not nearly as injurious as they would be if cooked. And they are excellent as fuel foods during the colder periods of the year. Their use in the warmer times of the year is unnecessary and ill-advised.

Summary of rating factors

1. 0 to 25. The food is rated according to its edibility and delectability in its fresh natural state.

2. 0 to minus (-) 100. The food is rated for its harmfulness in the human dietary. We should skirt as much as possible all foods that have within them unwelcome substances.

3. 0 to 25. The food is rated according to its digestibility and assimilability.

4. 0 to 50. The food is rated for its biological or nutritive value in human nutrition.

Food Rating Chart

For best health eat foods rated 80 or higher

NAME OF FOOD	RATING CRITERIA				TOTAL
	(1)	(2)	(3)	(4)	
ALMOND	22	-10	22	47	81
APPLE	25	0	25	42	92
APRICOT	25	0	25	46	96
APRICOT, Dried	20	0	20	40	80
AVOCADO	23	0	22	45	90
ASPARAGUS	15	-5	20	45	75
BANANA	25	0	25	48	98
BEAN, Green	22	0	25	47	94

BEAN, Sprouted & Greened in Sun

	20	0	23	47	90
BEET	15	-5	15	42	67
BERRIES (Generally)	23	0	25	45	93
BRAZIL NUT	23	0	23	47	93
BROCCOLI	24	0	25	47	96
BRUSSELS	22	0	24	46	92
CABBAGE	23	0	24	45	92
CANTALOUPES	25	0	25	47	97
CARROT	22	0	22	45	89
CASHEW	10	-5	15	45	65
CAULIFLOWER	23	0	25	45	93
CELERY	25	0	25	44	94
CHERIMOYA	25	0	25	45	95
CHERRY (Sweet)	25	0	25	45	95
COCONUT	20	-5	15	47	77
COLLARD GREENS	22	0	24	48	94
CORN (Fresh sweet)	25	0	25	45	95
CUCUMBER	20	0	20	40	80
CURRANT, Black	25	0	25	46	96
DANDELION	15	-25	15	48	53
DATE, Sun Dried	25	0	25	40	90
FIG (Fresh)	25	0	25	48	98
(Dried)	25	0	25	42	92
FILBERT (Hazel Nut)	22	0	23	47	92
GRAPES, (Generally)	25	0	25	47	97
GRAPEFRUIT	21	0	25	43	89
HONEYDEW MELON	25	0	25	47	97
KALE	23	0	23	48	94
LETTUCE, Romaine	25	0	25	45	95
Bibb	25	0	25	45	95
Iceberg	25	- 5	25	30	75
MANGO	25	0	25	47	97
MELONS (Generally)	25	0	25	41	97
OKRA	20	0	20	45	85
ORANGE	25	0	25	47	97

NAME OF FOOD	RATING CRITERIA				TOTAL
	(1)	**(2)**	**(3)**	**(4)**	
PAPAYA	25	0	25	47	97
PAW PAW	25	0	25	47	97
PEACH, Fresh	25	0	25	46	96
PEA, Fresh Green Sweet	25	0	25	46	96
PEANUT	12	-10	12	48	72
PEAR	25	0	25	45	95
PECAN	25	0	25	47	97
PEPITAS (Squash seeds)	20	0	25	47	92
PEPPER, Sweet Red	25	0	25	47	97
PINEAPPLE	25	0	25	47	97
PLUM	25	0	25	45	95
POTATO, Irish	5	0	20	45	70
POTATO, Sweet	15	0	20	45	80
RUTABAGA, Peeled	20	0	22	42	84
SESAME SEEDS	15	0	20	47	82
SPROUTS, Alfalfa, Mung, greened in the sun					
	20	0	23	47	90
SQUASH	25	-5	25	45	95
SUNFLOWER SEEDS	20	0	23	47	90
TANGERINE	25	0	25	45	95
TOMATO	25	0	25	45	95
TURNIP, Peeled	20	0	22	35	77
WALNUT	25	0	25	47	97
WATERMELON	25	0	25	45	95

8

Some Key Fruits
in a Natural Diet

Bananas: The Ideal Food For Humans

Bananas deserve the highest rank as food for humans. It is one of
the oldest foods of humans and has been treasured for its deliciousness. The ancients referred to the banana plant as the "Paradise Tree"
and its fruit as the fruit of paradise. Never has there been a more
apropos description of a food. Bananas are one of our most important foods and deserve a far greater role in our diet—in fact, they
should be our foremost item of diet as they are with many tropical
peoples, who also eat other tropical fruits such as breadfruit, jakfruit,
coconut, mango, etc. We are a class of frugivores that achieved our
high development with fruits of the tree as the bulk of our diet.
Fruits of the tree in our pristine habitat were mostly sweet fruits
such as bananas, figs, grapes and dates.

In its general suitability and beneficence in the human diet few
foods approach the banana. It is, ecologically and biologically, our
most ideal food. Dates, figs, grapes, melons and oranges, quite common foods, deserve a place in our diet but in the final analysis, the
banana wins on practically every count: economy, nutrition, convenience, plenitude, deliciousness, etc. Apples are a wholesome food
but they are woefully deficient in protein, having only 0.2% by
dry weight and then only two or three of the essential amino acids,
whereas bananas have all the essential amino acids and have about
5.2% protein dry weight.

Bananas are available all through the year. It is best to buy them
organically grown and green for ripening at home, where ripening
conditions can be controlled—you can try putting them in a brown
paper bag overnight, and expose them to air during the day. Commercially grown bananas are usually picked long before they are

ripe and nutritionally mature, and "gassed" with ethylene to facilitate ripening, as well as treated with such toxic chemicals as methyl bromide and aldicarb. Ethylene is the naturally occurring ripening gas produced by fruits; it is commercially synthesized by pyrolysis of hydrocarbons. Some organically grown bananas may also be gassed with ethylene, so your best odds of getting ungassed organic bananas may be to get them green. It also behooves you to ask your produce supplier if the bananas have been gassed, and to request ungassed organic bananas.

Select bananas free from surface bruises, with skin intact at both tips. Ripen at room temperature. When the skin is bright yellow speckled with brown, the starch has changed to fruit sugar, and the fruit will be tender sweet, and easy to digest. Fruit that ripens with brown speckles may not have been gassed, as I have been told that gassed bananas ripen with dark streaks and blotches instead of the brown speckles. I have found that speckled fruit is uniformly delightful in taste, so I am inclined to give some credence to this speculation.

I stress bananas as a major item in the diet primarily for reasons of overall goodness, availability and economy. It is of course beneficial to include other fruits as food, such as fresh figs, dates, grapes, or some other highly nutritious fruits, plus greens, some sea soft vegetables and nuts.

Humans are frugivores to their very cores! We'll do best if we respect our natural disposition. The banana is one of the ideal foods in the human diet.

* * *

Dates: The Fruit Of The Ages

by Todd Seliga

Possibly the first tree cultivated by humans, the enormous date palm yields a spectacular fruit. Dates require an extremely hot climate to flourish, at least 100 days of 100 degree Fahrenheit temperature. Temperatures during the summer and at the fall harvest exceed 120 degrees. This, along with their height, which averages 80 feet, makes harvesting no easy task since it means maneuvering 60 foot ladders and handling bunches of dates that weigh up to 60 pounds.

As I am a big date connoisseur and desert mystic, I visited my friends Jaime and Anjou Jones in Niland, California, prominent organic date farmers who have made quite a reputation for themselves growing superb dates in the Southern California desert. Now calling themselves "The Date People," Jaime started out farming his own dates in 1985 under the name "Cahuilla Gardens." Jaime, a twelve year raw foodist, is one of the few date farmers known as a "palmero" for his ability to work the tall date palms and maneuver a 62 foot date ladder. Being a raw foodist makes it much easier to work in these extreme desert temperatures and to keep up with the strenuous demands of farming dates throughout the entire year.

The Date People's present name emerged in 1990 when Anjou met Jaime and came to work for his blossoming operation. Jaime celebrated his twentieth year of full-time agricultural work this past August. Of these 20 years, 19 have been on organic farms since Jaime was unable to find work on an organic farm during his first year.

Jaime began Cahuilla Gardens in 1985 with little more than a bicycle and a lot of motivation and energy while maintaining a day job. He worked this leased grove into a reputable business that provided him with a living. By 1990 he and Anjou were working several groves and employing many migrant and alternative workers during harvesting time (September to November). The Date People point to an enormous community feeling amongst workers on their farm. It is not uncommon for many who have gone on to do other things over the years to visit now and again.

Nineteen ninety-eight marked another great accomplishment for the Date People when Jaime and Anjou moved to Niland, California, purchasing their own land. Niland, once dubbed the "winter" Tomato Capital of the world, is now characterized by The Date

People's newly planted date grove of over 500 date palm shoots. Moving from their leased grove in Borrego Springs, Jaime and Anjou still maintain some groves in Coachella Valley.

The new grove in Niland is a magnificent sight amidst beautiful desert scenery and clearly the product of tremendous work. Desert flowers and shrubs abound and delight anyone wandering through them. The dry desert rocky terrain of the Chocolate Mountains off to the east can be seen, with its sculpted beauty. Jaime's genuine enthusiasm for dates reveals itself in the fruits of his grove. I have known few people so motivated and dedicated to their work.

None of their farm work comes at any cost to the environment or to the health and well-being of the harvesters. Jaime chooses to have his groves certified only by the most stringent organic certifier, Oregon Tilth Certified Organic. The Date People's processed dates (date rolls and nuggets) are unique in that they are raw, having been spared the industry standard of cooking using steam hydration. Anjou and Jaime process their soft dates instead of the drier Deglet Noor date (which are commonly used and almost always requires steam hydration). The soft dates retain their enzymes making them easier to digest than their store bought (cooked) counterparts. This makes it extremely important to buy dates and processed date products directly from a grower who can assure you they are not hydrated.

As well as the traditional sugary sweet Medjhool and the nutty Deglet Noor, there are over 140 kinds of dates in the world. Barhis, Zahidis, black dates, Halawis, and Borrego Honeys are the names of only a few.

Dates can be enjoyed fresh and whole, processed into nuggets or rolls, or even blended with water or fruit juice into smoothies. Dates are best known in their dried form. However, each year's harvest brings to market a significant number of undried dates in their fresh moist form. Moist dates are by far the absolute best. They literally melt in one's mouth and can be relished in quantity due to their extreme moistness. Being very moist their sugars are less concentrated and they digest like high water content fruit.

Drying preserves the fruit's shelf life. This may be done by using fans or through natural drying on the trees as practiced by The Date People. The fan simply draws the moisture out without any heat being involved.

The hardiest palms yield 500 or more pounds of fruit. In their newsletter, *The International Dateline*, Anjou and Jaime note: "One date palm planted at birth could conceivably supply a person with practically their entire lifetime supply of food." Dates are almost nutritionally complete and are a food staple in north Africa and the Middle East.

Human history reveals a long acquaintance with dates. Mentioned in the Bible, spoken of in Eastern poetry, and uncovered in archaeological finds, the date palm enjoys a long and uninterrupted relationship with humankind. Today's leading producers are Iraq and Egypt, but dates also abound in Saudi Arabia, Iran, Algeria, Pakistan, and Sudan. Nearly all of the United States' dates come from Arizona's Salt River and the Colorado River Valley near Yuma along with the Salton Basin and interior valleys of California.

Female date palms produce fruit while the males produce the pollen. One male tree can produce enough pollen for fifty females. Date growers must do the pollination by hand, collecting and carrying the pollen to the female flowers. The fruit develops following pollination and remains green and bitter, resembling an olive, before turning yellow or red, and finally ripening into shades of gold, brown, or black. Date palms begin to fruit anywhere from four to ten years following their planting, and flourish in sandy alkaline soil. The main necessity for date cultivation, of course, is water for irrigation. Date bunches are susceptible to damage when nearing ripeness and are bagged or netted to prevent water, bird, or insect damage.

It is crucial when purchasing this sweet oblong fruit to make sure it is organically grown, or grown using similar practices. As The Date People explain, organic dates, as compared to non-organic dates, provide "more nutrition, better taste, [are part of a] healthier lifestyle, are not exposed to "malathion-insecticide, methyl bromide-fumigant, chlorine solutions-mold inhibitor, [nor do they cause] a more toxic environment." Commercial dates harm both our health and the life sustaining ability of their bioregion.

Date harvesting is a complicated and timely process. Dates need to be picked at exactly the right time when neither too wet (if harvested early) nor too dry (if harvested late). If the dates are too wet they are prone to damage when being handled and may mold when kept in storage. Dates which are too dry have less flavor and more chance of becoming bug-infested.

The harvested dates are usually minimally dried and stored in refrigeration making them readily available year round.

Dates are a nourishing addition to our diets. They can be enjoyed and relied upon for availability throughout the year. With so many diverse varieties to be had at such reasonable prices, dates can be easily stored and refrigerate well for over a year from their harvest. With the fast pace of life, they are a convenient and nutritious food source which also brings one great pleasure.

Date Nutrition Facts*

(based on a serving of 10 dates, 85 grams edible portion)

Calories	240
Carbohydrate	57 g
Dietary Fiber	6.4 g
Potassium	560 mg
Protein	2 g
Fat	0 g
Sodium	9 mg

Ten dates provide the following percentages of the U.S. Recommended Daily Allowances (USRDA) for these nutrients:

Protein	4
Thiamin (Vitamin B1)	2
Riboflavin (Vitamin B2)	6
Niacin	6
Calcium	4
Iron	4

Vitamin B6	8
Folic Acid	4
Phosphorus	4
Magnesium	10
Zinc	2
Copper	6
Pantothenic Acid	4

*Source: California Date Administrative Committee Nutrition Analysis (Hazelton Laboratories of America Inc., May, 1997.)

Editor's note: It is assumed that the analyzed dates were not organically grown. From this and other analyses, dates appear to be one of the most nutrient rich foods on the planet. The USRDA statistics are provided only as a benchmark; USRDA's are derived from conventional standard American cooked food dietetics based on an unhealthy population and are of little real value in many regards; USRDA theory falls apart when we study raw food nutritional science.

* * *

Kiwis: Treasures With a Split Personality

by David Klein

Shaped like a goose egg and deviously disguised in a fuzzy skin resembling a plain brown wrapper, kiwi fruits seem like one of nature's best kept secret treasures. Their dull outer appearance belies the sensual magnificence within.

Kiwis are the fruit of vining plants which beautifully adorn many patio fences and canopies in Northern California, the home of Living Nutrition. The fruits mature and drop in the coldest months of the year. They will be slightly soft when ripe and easy to peel. Avoid those which are very soft or mushy—they are over-ripe and bland at best. If you have never tried a fresh, perfectly ripe kiwi, brace yourself! Inside is a delicious tangy lime-green pulp which will energize (or should I say jolt?) the senses.

Tiny black seeds bespeckle this green flesh, adding a subtle, slightly crunchy pizzazz of their own. The green flesh envelops a sweet, creamy pith which, although only a bite sized morsel, is a lemony-banana flavored treasure unto itself...a little slice of Heaven.

The contrasting tanginess and mellowness of the inner and outer parts make kiwi eating a most Quixotic experience! There are few fruits that can match its duality of flavors and textures. Just the anticipation of the next bite can bamboozle the brain waves, but the fulfillment is an unforgettable delight.

Then there is the added dimension of the visual show. Bite or slice one in half and gaze at its cross-section. The splendid symmetry, rich colors and opulent design may remind one of a supernatural cat's eye. Or...? Write in and let us know what you see!

As if the exquisite taste sensations were not enough, kiwis rank with dates and bananas as the most nutritionally complete foods on the planet. Peeled by hand and eaten mono, or sliced and eaten in salads, kiwis are many things to the senses and exceptionally good for the body.

California Kiwifruit Nutritional Values*

A serving of California Kiwifruit has more dietary fiber than a bowl of bran flakes, twice the vitamin C of an orange or grapefruit, and ounce for ounce as much potassium as a banana. Serving size: 2 typical peeled, 5.3 oz.

Calories	90
Sodium	0 mg
Protein	1 g
Potassium	450 mg
Cholesterol	0 grams
Dietary Fiber	4 g
Carbohydrates	18 g
Fat	1 g

	% USRDA**
Protein	2%
Vitamin E	10%
Vitamin A	2%
Vitamin B6	4%
Vitamin C	230%
Folacin	8%
Phosphorus	2%
Riboflavin	2%
Magnesium	6%
Niacin	2%
Copper	8%
Calcium	4%
Pantothenic Acid	2%
Iron	4%

*Source: California Kiwifruit Commission
**USRDA's are provided for relative comparison only.

* * *

Avocado:
The Fruit That Would Make
Butter and Meat Obsolete

by David Klein

If you love fatty, creamy, hearty foods and want to avoid the choles-terol and toxicity of meat and dairy, anchor your diet with avocado!

Avocado is more than just a tasty treat to be enjoyed in guacamole—it makes a hearty satisfying meal when eaten alone, in salads, and in other dishes. Most people who transition from a stan-dard American diet to a vegan diet with avocado, nuts and seeds don't miss the animal foods because raw vegan plant fat is so satisfying as well as more nutritious than cooked fatty animal foods! In hundreds of thousands of cases, people who've adopted a vegan diet of predominantly raw foods with minimal or no cooked starches as part of a healthful lifestyle (including regular exercise and adequate sleep), have lost excess weight, overcome illness, gained new vitality, and avoided the killer diseases which now plague our meat, bread, dairy, and junk-food eating society. The fresh vitamins, active enzymes, organic minerals, soluble fiber, high water content, and easily digested fats and proteins in avocados and other fruit and plant foods can help transform any sluggish, overweight meat eater into a slimmer and more dynamic person. Some of the leanest people I know eat the most avocados! Cooked foods such as bread, pasta, meat, dairy and junk foods are the villains that can keep an avocado eater from losing excess fat.

If your goal is to reduce your consumption or transition completely off of meat and dairy, avocado may be the perfect way to satisfy your natural cravings for creamy nourishment. Dr. William Esser writes in his *Dictionary of Natural Foods*:

"The avocado is one of the most valuable foods which nature has given man. For those concerned about eliminating meat from their diet, this offers not merely a "substitute," but a food which is much superior in value for human maintenance. It is rich in protein and fat and comparatively higher than any other fruits in these elements. The fat is more digestible than animal fats."

Avocado is also known as the "alligator pear" because of the rough skin on some varieties. In the 17th and 18th centuries the fruit was also commonly known as "butter pear." In tropical Central America, avocado trees have been growing wild for thousands of years, providing natives with a rich food. The Aztecs called the tree Ahuacatl. Marauding Spanish armies changed this to abocado or avocado, the now common English name.

According to the *Little Green Avocado Book*, there is strong evidence that avocado trees flourished 50 million years ago in what is now California, and avocados might have provided food for dinosaurs.

106

Today's avocados are derived from three natural races. The Mexican type (semi-tropical) produces small fruits, 6 to 10 ounces having glossy purple, paper-thin skin when ripe. The Guatemalan type (subtropical) yields medium pear-shaped fruits which are first green, turning purple-black or coppery-purple when ripe, with a typically tough shell. The West Indian type (tropical) produces enormous, smooth, round, glossy green fruits as up to 2 pounds in weight. In the United States, 95 percent of the commercially grown avocados come from California, with small percentages coming from Florida, Louisiana, Texas and Hawaii. The *California Rare Fruit Growers Fruit Facts, Volume One*, reports that avocados grow well in valley and coastal California, as far north as Cape Mendocino and Red Bluff. Hybrid forms of all types are grown.

Avocado growing is relatively new in the United States. They are available year round. The harvest time depends on the variety. The Hass, the best known commercial variety, is a hybrid of the Mexican and the Guatemalan types and is picked from January into fall depending on where it is grown.

The *Little Green Avocado Book* also reports that avocado trees are large evergreens of the laurel family, and there are about 400 commercial varieties of avocado. Some are: Bacon, Ettinger, Fuerte, Gwen, Hass, Nabal, Pinkerton, Reed and Zutano. Mexican types ripen in 6 to 8 months from bloom, Guatemalan types 12 to 18 months.

There are wide differences in the flavors of individual avocados, ranging from salty, to nutty, to sweet, with shades in between. If a fruit has been picked too early it may be watery and unpalatable. If picked too late, some varieties develop a rancid flavor. If a Bacon avocado tastes like bacon, it is rancid. If an avocado has dark flesh (rot), compost it and/or salvage the good parts.

At some farmers markets and produce stores, one can occasionally find "Cukes" (also known as "Cocktail" or "Finger" avocados), seedless, pickle-shaped avocado fruits which result from improperly pollinated flowers. One can also occasionally find miniature avocados which have thin, black edible skin and an anise flavor (the Mexicola is one variety)—these make a delightful treat!

Julie Frink, Curator for the Avocado Variety Collection, University of California Research Station at Irvine, California, writes:

"I have nearly 20 varieties growing in my yard and the Hass variety is always one of the best. Some of the green varieties sold in stores have given a bad name to some really fine green skinned fruits. The most inferior tasting avocados have either been picked when too immature or they are poor quality pollinator varieties to begin with. One of our favorites is the round, green Reed. A perfect Reed on Labor Day is a most fantastic treat! So often these wonderful fall avocados are picked and sold in the spring when they are watery and tasteless. The green, elongated pear shaped Pinkerton can be fantastic if allowed to stay on the tree until full maturity but will be rubbery and tasteless if picked too soon."

The *Little Green Avocado Book* also states that an acre of avocado trees can yield more food than an acre of any other tree crop. Imagine the ecological implications—a perfectly healthful "meaty" food which requires 1/200th or less of the acreage needed by the cattle industry for a comparable yield in pounds, posing no pollution problems—and no carnage! Worried about mad cow disease?—eat raw avocados, seeds and nuts and stay sane and mentally keen!

Avocados are bursting with nutrients—vitamins A, B-complex, C, E, H, K, and folic acid, plus the minerals magnesium, copper, iron, calcium, potassium and many other trace elements. Avocados provide all of the essential amino acids (those that must be provided by our diet), with 18 amino acids in all, plus 7 fatty acids, including Omega 3 and 6. Avocados contain more protein than cow's milk, about 2% per edible portion. Since rapidly growing nursing infants obtain no more than 2% protein from mother's milk, we can safely assume that children and adults do not regularly require foods richer in protein than avocado. Our bodies recycle approximately 80% of our protein; cooked protein is denatured and largely unusable, thus our protein need is far lower than what is taught by conventional dietetics. A small avocado will provide more usable protein then a huge steak because cooked protein in meat is deranged and mostly unavailable to our liver, the organ which makes all of our body's protein. There is clear evidence from many sources that cooked fatty and high-protein foods are the prime culprit in our country's high rate of cancer, as well as in colitis, Crohn's disease and many other diseases. (I instantly healed up from a long illness, ulcerative colitis, seventeen years ago after I stopped eating meat and adopted a properly combined low-fat vegan diet of mostly raw fruits and vegetables, and I have since helped over 1,000 people recover from similar illnesses). Ripe, raw organically grown avocados are naturally pure and furnish all of the elements we need to build the highest quality protein in our bodies.

The water content of avocado by weight averages 74%. Because avocado is a ripe, watery, enzymatically-alive fruit, it ranks as the most easily digested rich source of fats and proteins in whole food form. The ripening action of the sun "predigests" complex proteins into simple, easily digested amino acids. The fat content (by weight) varies from 7 to 26 % according to the variety, averaging 15%. Approximately 63% of the fat in avocados is monounsaturated, 20% is polyunsaturated and 17% is saturated. Avocados are the perfect source of dietary fat—appetizing in their raw state, digestible, and pure. Another plus is that avocados have no cholesterol.

Avocado is an alkalinizing food, i.e., the mineral end products of metabolism have an alkalinizing effect in the blood and other bodily fluids. Because the human body works to maintain a slightly alkaline pH, an alkalinizing diet is the most healthful way of eating. Meat, dairy and most raw nuts create acidity in the body— excess eating of these causes the leaching of alkalinizing calcium from our bones to buffer the acidity, leading to osteoporosis. Dr. Douglas Graham states:

"Current bone density testing has verified loss of calcium from the bones after the consumption of just one meat meal. A similar meal containing the same amount of protein from plants results in no calcium loss. Fruit and vegetable proteins, which supply the complete spectrum of human nutrients, must be considered superior to animal protein which are deficient or missing many of our essential nutrients such as fiber, vitamin C and a host of phytonutrients and antioxidants."

Avocado eaters who eat a healthful vegan diet typically experience more lustrous hair, softer, smoother skin, more pliable nails, fewer joint problems, slimmer belly, less body odor, improved mental function and enhanced libido. Upon giving up animal meat and dairy, switching to a diet of 75% to 100% raw vegan foods with enzymatically-alive "plant meat," and adopting a healthful lifestyle, a multitude of people have reaped amazing health benefits and joyous vitality.

How to eat avocado

The natural way - Using your claws (fingernails), peel off the skin. The skin of a naturally ripened avocado will easily spiral off in one to three pieces. Try this: slide a whole nude avocado through your lips and eat it slowly. There is no more sensual eating experience!

The modern way - Using a knife, slice an avocado along the north-south or east-west axis, then remove the pit. The halves can be sliced into smaller segments. The skin can then be peeled off, or you can scoop out the flesh with a spoon. Eat plain as a snack or scoop the flesh into a bowl or onto a salad.

Avocado generally requires approximately one and a half to two hours in the stomach to be digested. It digests well if the eater is relaxed, hungry, energetic, has an empty stomach and follows proper food combining guidelines. If one eats avocado when tired, one may fall asleep.

For optimum digestion, eat avocado alone or with any non-sweet-non-starchy fruit or any non-starchy vegetable food. Eating avocado with leafy greens, celery and/or cucumber will enhance the digestive process as additional digestive enzymes are secreted. People with weak digestion will generally experience enhanced digestion when eating avocado with non-starchy salads as opposed to eating avocado alone.

Avoid eating avocado with or within 20 minutes of eating sweet fruit or drinking sweet fruit juice. The combination of little bit of lemon or grapefruit juice with avocado tends to digest well for most people.

Wait at least 3 hours after eating avocado before eating sweet fruit.

Do not eat avocado with any other kind of oily, fatty or high-protein food such as seeds, nuts, coconut, olives, yogurt, cream, cheese or meat. Wait several hours between eating these foods, although the ideal is 24 hours. It takes several hours to digest and utilize any kind of heavy/oily food, and the body can only digest one at a time

Some people become sluggish and do not function well when eating heavy foods in the morning; it might be best to eat avocado mid-day and after.

Avoid eating avocado if you are experiencing acid reflux, indigestion, sore throat, inflammation or fever.

Overeating avocados can lead to sluggishness, hyper-acid stomach, and skin outbreaks.

The quantity of avocados that is healthful for you is a function of your taste preferences and digestion. Generally, one a day, three to six days per week is a good baseline. For best results, tune in to your body's senses and observe your energy levels, digestion and elimination.

Avocado preparation ideas

Transition
• Mash avocado ("avo butter") into baked potatoes.
• Smear "avo butter" over steamed vegetables.
• Dollop warmed "avo butter" over hot air popped corn.
• Spread "avo butter" on whole grain bread and soft corn tortillas
• Dip baked corn chips into a avo halves, or a bowl of avo pulp.
All raw
• Halve and pit avocado then scoop (or "dip") celery, carrot, broccoli, bell pepper pieces in and eat as a snack
• Add to salads—there's your dressing!

- Mix with chopped bell pepper, tomato, celery, lemon juice, etc. for guacamole or salsa.
- Party time: slice into spears or chunks, insert toothpicks, and serve as hors d'oeuvres. (Who needs cholesterol and fat laden cheese!?)
- Make veggie "handwiches" or "veggie roll-ups"—place chopped veggies, sprouts, tomatoes and avocado chunks on lettuce, or kale or cabbage leaves, fold them over or roll them up, and enjoy.
- Add to processed vegetables—veggie slaw, veggie loafs, veggie cakes and cookies.
- Mix into veggie and sprout soups—blend in to make a creamy texture, or serve "chunky style."
- Make dressings—avo-carrot juice, avo-tomato-celery (add a little lemon or grapefruit juice and/or herbs to taste).
- "Avo butter"—smear a halved avocado over freshly shucked corn on the cob
- "Avo butter"—spread avocado on Essene (sprouted grain) crackers.
- Stuff avocado and veggies into cored bell peppers (whole or halved) and serve as a "handwich" or other entrée.

Note: avocado and starchy foods (e.g., potatoes, bread, grains, corn, old carrots) make a "fair" food combination—for optimal digestion, do not combine avocado and starchy foods.

Some extraordinary avocado uses

House Plants - Stick toothpicks in the sides of avocado pits and set them on the top of a water-filled glass. A plant will sprout forth which can be transplanted into a pot after a few weeks. On the Avocado Information Web Site, University of California, Cooperative Extension, Dr. Mary Lu Arpaia and Dr. Ben Faber report:

"It is possible to grow an avocado from seed, just don't let it dry out. Be aware that the seed is the result of cross-pollination so the resulting tree will be different from the tree the fruit came from. For example, if you plant the seed from a Hass avocado, the resulting tree will be a cross between a Hass and something else... it will

NOT be a Hass! Also, keep in mind that avocados planted from seed take anywhere from 5 to 13 years+ before they flower and produce fruit. When I start an avocado from seed I usually take it right from the fruit, I cut about 1/4" off the tip of the seed with a sharp knife, and place the seed in a pot with potting soil with just the flat/cut top of the seed showing above the soil. Keep it moist and wait...(time to germinate varies)."

Hand cream - If you have chapped hands or want to prevent chapping in the winter, rub in some avocado.

Shaving cream - Smear it on!

Sunburn relief - It may not block any of the sun but it will help keep your skin moist.

Foot and hand massage - With your partner, share the luxury of a relaxing massage. If you both have sex in mind, don't stop at the hands and feet!

Avocado vs. animal meat

Avocado - Watery and fiber-rich, non-consiptating.
Animal Meat - Low water, no fiber constipating.

Avocado - Has all essential amino acids.
Animal Meat - Amino acids denatured by cooking.

Avocado - No cholesterol.
Animal Meat - High in cholesterol.

Avocado - Takes 2 to 4 hours to digest, normally will not putrefy.
Animal Meat - Takes 12 to 24 hours to digest, normally putrefies, poisoning our blood, tissues and brain.

Avocado - No parasites, pathogens or tumors.
Animal Meat - Incidences of parasites, pathogens and tumors range from rare to common.

Avocado - Not inoculated with any chemicals.

Animal Meat - Typically inoculated with antibiotics, medicines and hormones.

Avocado - Water-rich and non-allergenic.
Animal Meat - Bloody and laden with allergenic proteins.

Avocado - Does not need cooking or any preparation other than peeling.
Animal Meat - If eaten raw, the parasite-pathogen risk increases; when cooked the fats become carcinogenic, the proteins coagulate, and the heat-deaminated minerals become embedded as arterial and bowel plaque leading to atherosclerosis, heart disease, Alzeimer's, etc.

Avocado - 100% healthful.
Animal Meat - A major health hazard with links to cancer, colitis, diabetes, obesity and many other diseases.

Avocado - Alkalizing.
Animal Meat - Acidifying.

Avocado - The fuel required to digest avocado and other fruity fats is less than half of that required to digest meats, and digestion time is dramatically lower as well.
Animal Meat - Takes approximately 50% of body's energy and as much as three days to digest and clean up the toxins from its decomposition in the gut and the immune system response to the toxic proteins and grease which enter the blood.

Avocado - 100% ecologically sound.
Animal Meat - Ecologically destructive, requiring up to 200 times the acreage and over 10 times the quantity of water to produce one pound of food (approximately 220 gallons of water per pound of avocado vs. 2,400 gallons water per pound of beef); grazing causes soil erosion and in some countries deforestation; liquid, solid and gaseous animal wastes pollute the atmosphere, land and waterways.

114

Some avocado myths and facts

Myth - It's a vegetable.
Fact - It's actually an oily berry—a fruit.

Myth - It's high in cholesterol.
Fact - It has no cholesterol. Only animal foods have cholesterol.

Myth - It's high in fat.
Fact - By weight, avocados average 30% easily digestible oily fatty acids and approximately 70% water.

Myth - Its saturated fat content is dangerous.
Fact - Only about 2.5% of the edible portion of avocado is saturated fat, and unheated saturated fat from live plant foods is non-toxic.

Myth - It's fattening.
Fact - It is the cooked starches, meat, dairy and processed sugar in people's diets that feed their fat cells. Most active people who consume avocados as part high raw food vegan diet have no problem losing excess fat and staying lean.

Myth - It is a tree ripened fruit.
Fact - The avocado doesn't soften on the tree. After dropping or picking it must be allowed to soften for 4 to 17 days depending on the variety and ambient temperature and humidity.

Myth - It is best to ripen it in a bag.
Fact - Not necessary. Keep your weekly supply of avocados on your kitchen table, counter or somewhere else in plain sight. Pinch the tops and bottoms each morning and when they yield to pressure on both ends they are ripe. Refrigerate the ones you are not ready to eat.

Myth - It can't be refrigerated.

Fact - Yes it can. Wrap ripe avocado in plastic or keep it in a plastic bag or container. If it is refrigerated for too long some spoiling may result. Remove unripened avocado from the refrigerator 2 or 3 days before you intend to eat them.

Myth - Keep the seed in to keep the guacamole from turning black.
Fact - That is an old wives tale! Wrap it in plastic to keep oxidation at bay.

References

Arpaia, Dr. Mary Lu and Faber, Dr. Ben. *Answers to Questions.* Avocado Information Web Site, University of California, Cooperative Extension.
http://ucavo.ucr.edu/General/Answers.html#anchor417098.
California Avocado Commission. www.avocado.org.
California Rare Fruit Growers Inc. *Fruit Facts, Volume One.* Fullerton, CA: Fullerton Arboretum, CSUF,1992.
The Committee on Diet, Nutrition and Cancer. *Diet, Nutrition and Cancer.* Washington, D.C.: National Academy Press, 1982.
Doeser, Linda. *The Little Green Avocado Book.* New York, NY: St. Martin's Press, 1981.
Esser, Dr. William. *Dictionary of Natural Foods.* Bridgeport, CT: Natural Hygiene Press, 1972.
Ford Heritage. *Composition and Facts About Foods.* Pomeroy, WA: Health Research, 1971.
Fry, T. C., Vetrano, Dr. Vivian V., et. al. *The Life Science Health System.* Austin, TX: Life Science Institute, 1986.
Robbins, John. *The Diet Revolution.* Berkeley, CA: Conari Press, 2001.
Shelton, Dr. Herbert M. *Food Combining Made Easy.* San Antonio, TX: Willow Publishing, Inc., 1982.
USDA Nutrient Database for Standard Reference, Release 13, November, 1999. www.nal.usda.gov.
Wai. *New Substances In Prepared Food.* www.23.waisays.com.

9
Dietary Transition
by David Klein

How does one begin as they change to a diet of increasingly raw foods? My advice to people desiring success on the raw food path is that they first get a proper education in nutrition and self-healing from Dr. Shelton's, Dr. T. C. Fry's, Dr. Douglas Graham's and Arthur Baker's books, and second, that they tune in to their bodies' signals to discern what they truly need for nourishment, balance and healing. Here are some guidelines on how to make the transition to a diet of 90% to 100% alive raw organic foods.

From SAD to RAW

Phase 1 - Immediately to 3 weeks

• Discontinue salt.
• Go vegan: phase out all meat, eggs and dairy—replace with avocado, nuts and seeds.
• Discontinue white bread, white rice and soy products.
• Replace white bread with whole brain bread or avoid all bread entirely.
• Discontinue processed cheese.
• Discontinue all soft drinks and caffeinated beverages.
• Phase out all junk foods.
• Replace processed sugar sweets with dried and fresh fruit and raw honey.
• Begin shopping at healthfood stores, buying fruits and vegetables.
• Begin following food combining: fruit alone or with green vegetables; avoid eating starches with high protein foods.
• Have some fruit for breakfast—try citrus—and vegetable salads with each cooked food meal.
• Use a steamer to cook.

- Drink several glasses of distilled water per day, mostly in the morning.
- Exercise vigorously at least once per day.
- Optional: begin experimenting with fresh made fruit and vegetable juices.

Phase 2 - 3 to 8 weeks

- Have only raw food for breakfast, and no cooked food till noon (if at all).
- Phase out all pasta and white flour products.
- Phase out whole grain bread, cereals and related products.
- Gradually increase your raw food intake to at least 75%.
- Have nuts/seeds only once per day (if at all).
- Do not eat starchy foods on the same day of eating nuts/seeds.

Phase 3 - 6 weeks to as long as it takes

- Gradually increase your raw food consumption to 90% to 100%.
- Follow proper food combining all of the time.

Food shopping tips

- Experiment—try new foods.
- Get in touch with the foods your body finds to be most flavorful or refreshing and observe and select the most fragrant and visually attractive foods.
- Don't over-stock perishable foods—shop often.
- Buy your mainstays in bulk quantities.
- Go 100% organic.
- Frequent farmer's markets if available.

Dietary transition meal ideas

Follow your taste buds and other senses. Only eat and drink what tastes delicious or refreshing. Eat lightly in the morning. Eat no more than one heavy meal per day, unless you are engaged in heavy activity. If you are eating cooked food, always have a bigger portion of raw vegetables with it. Work at eating only when you are truly hungry—become aware of emotional and other habitual eating patterns. Practice mindfulness as you select, prepare and chew your food. Remember that simple is best, and work on any overeating tendencies. If sweet fruit is appealing but make you feel unbalanced, minimize the sweet fruit while eating it with cucumbers, celery and/or greens—or do a citrus and vegetable juice and water cleanse to clean out and improve your digestion. If you have strong cravings for fat and want to eat lots or nuts or avocado, or strong cravings for starch and want to eat lots of cooked starchy foods, have some of those foods if that feels right, however have plenty of cucumbers, celery and/or greens with them. Bring your healthful food with you to the workplace and when you travel.

Sample breakfast meal choices

• Fresh orange or grapefruit juice (wait 20 minutes after drinking), bananas, cucumber, lettuce.
• Oranges, mandarins, peaches or nectarines with celery or cucumber.
• Melon (eat alone). optional: followed 20 minutes later by bananas and celery.
• Berries, apples, dates, celery.
• Apple-celery juice-banana smoothie.

Sample lunch and dinner choices

No more than one raw-with-cooked food meal per day is recommended.

• Garden salad with tomatoes, avocado and rinsed dulse leaf.
Optional: carrot juice-avocado dressing.

• Garden salad with cucumber, tomato and raw or germinated seeds or nuts.
Optional: cucumber-grapefruit juice dressing.

• Garden salad with sunflower greens (sprouts).
Optional: carrot-avocado dressing.
Optional: fresh lemon juice dressing.
Optional: seed "cheese"-dill-lemon dressing.

• Seed or almond "cheese."
Celery, cucumber and greens.

• Juicy carrot-broccoli pulp (from a juicer) with avocado mashed in.
Celery, cucumber, rinsed dulse leaf.

• Grated vegetables with avocado "mayonnaise."
• Garden salad with celery and avocado.
Transition choices: steamed broccoli, yams, sweet potato, squash,
beets, turnips, asparagus, cabbage.

• Garden salad with raw corn and avocado.
Transition choices: baked potato with avocado "butter."

• Garden salad with raw corn and avocado.
Transition choices: soft corn tortilla "buttered" with avocado and
filled with raw and steamed vegetables.

See Chapter 13 - Alive Raw Food Recipes for more ideas.

Healthful snacks

Avocado, dates, raisins, figs, apples, pears, oranges, nuts and
seeds (raw or soaked 12 to 36 hours), fruit smoothies, banana "ice
cream," carrot juice, coconut water. Transition: popcorn with avocado "butter," baked, saltless corn chips with raw salsa.

Try 100% raw one day!

You can do it! Juicing can help you get ready. Don't force it.
Don't judge yourself. Follow your loftiest goals, let it flow and enjoy!

10
Healthful Eating Guidelines
by David Klein

• Eat only if you are hungry.
• Exercise to create true hunger, especially before breakfast.
• Do not eat when tired or emotionally upset.
• Drink one or more glasses of purified water before breakfast.
• Biologically, we are frugivores. Fruit is our natural and most health-ful food. A diet of 50% to 90% fruit (by weight—sweet and non-sweet) is recommended.
• Include plenty of cucumbers, tomatoes (both are botanically clas-sified as fruits), celery and leafy greens in your diet.
• The most healthful food choices are raw/living fruits, vegetables and sprouts with minimal amounts of seeds, and nuts, all fresh from the orchard and garden.
• Eat fruit for breakfast.
• Learn how to tune into your body's hunger signals toward eating instinctively. Sniff your food before eating. If the sensation is plea-surable, you are ready to eat; if you do not receive a pleasurable sensation, that food will generally not be nourishing for you at that time—try other foods or inquire into whether you are truly hungry.
• Eat only fresh food that tastes delicious.
• Do not drink more than a few sips of juices or water when eating solid food.
• Chew your food slowly and well. Mix the food with your saliva. Chew solid food until thoroughly liquefied.
• While eating, if the experience or food becomes unappealing or you feel satisfied, stop eating; do not overeat.
• Follow food combining guidelines to a "t." Eat fruit only on an empty stomach. Eat melons alone. Eat citrus fruits before sweet fruits. Do not eat fatty/protein foods (seeds and nuts, including coconut) with sweet fruit or starchy foods (squash, tubers, carrots

and corn). Legumes are poorly digested and not recommended; sprouted legumes are somewhat more digestible, yet are of marginal value. Protein/fatty foods, starchy foods and legumes all combine well with all vegetables and non-sweet fruits. Do not mix tomatoes with starchy foods. Avocado combines well with any kind of vegetable, tuber and non-sweet fruit.

• Avoid old rancid nuts and seeds. Living nuts and seeds germinated in water for 12 to 24 hours are more digestible than ungerminated (raw) ones.

• Space out your meals to allow time for your food to digest. Fruit digests within minutes. Starches require about two to four hours. Protein foods require about four to six hours.

• Cultivate self-awareness about your eating, plan out your food choices and eat consciously and only when relaxed.

• Eat only organically or biodynamically grown foods.

• Do not eat within two hours of going to sleep.

• Make a gradual transition off of all cooked food.

• If during your transition you are eating cooked food, never eat a meal of all cooked food; always eat a bigger portion of raw food with the cooked food.

• The most healthful cooked foods are steamed vegetables, squash and potatoes. Cooked grains are not recommended—they are sedating, mucus-forming and constipating.

• Avoid or eat minimally of hot, spicy and irritating "foods" such as curries, spices, black pepper, onions, radishes, mustard greens, garlic and chili peppers.

• Avoid all animal products (all animal flesh, eggs and dairy), heated oils, chemical additives and preservatives, salt, spices, flour, white rice, white sugar, coffees, caffeinated teas, pasteurized drinks, irradiated foods, non-organic and non-whole foods and supplements, fermented products, roasted seeds and nuts, caramelized and crystallized dried sweet fruits, chlorinated and fluoridated water, and drugs.

• Learn how to inquire inwardly to understand the meaning of any emotional eating habits and cravings. Get the right guidance.

• Eat to support your body's efforts to create excellent health. Eat for bodily purity, perfect digestion, mental clarity, consistent balanced energy, and high vitality.

• If you are going to a place where healthful food will not be available, bring your own.

• Do not place any healing faith in food. Food has no healing power. Your body has all of the healing power.

• If you are ill, ingest only purified water and fresh juices—do not eat any heavy foods, such as seeds and nuts. Get the right healing guidance.

• Choose to live and eat healthfully.

• Each day affirm that your dietary transition is an unfolding process that will improve your life in wonderful ways, and give yourself the patience and nurturing love you deserve.

• Stay on the raw food path for life. Don't allow anyone to influence you waywardly.

• Share your life with other health-minded supportive friends.

• Get the right education and guidance. Study books by Dr. Herbert Shelton on food combining, nutrition and fasting.

• Eat to live; don't live to eat. Find many daily pleasurable activities to enjoy; don't allow your life to revolve around food.

The Raw Food Pearamid

by David Klein

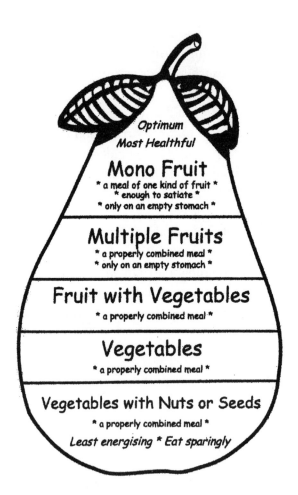

Optimum
Most Healthful

Mono Fruit
* a meal of one kind of fruit *
* enough to satiate *
* only on an empty stomach *

Multiple Fruits
* a properly combined meal *
* only on an empty stomach *

Fruit with Vegetables
* a properly combined meal *

Vegetables
* a properly combined meal *

Vegetables with Nuts or Seeds
* a properly combined meal *
*Least energising * Eat sparingly*

Food Combining Chart

by David Klein, derived from Life Science

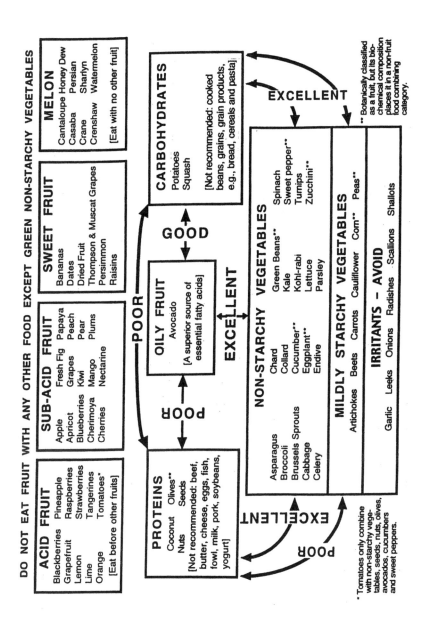

DO NOT EAT FRUIT WITH ANY OTHER FOOD EXCEPT GREEN NON-STARCHY VEGETABLES

ACID FRUIT

Blackberries Pineapple
Grapefruit Raspberries
Lemon Strawberries
Lime Tangerines
Orange Tomatoes*

[Eat before other fruits]

SUB-ACID FRUIT

Apple Fresh Fig Papaya
Apricot Grapes Peach
Blueberries Kiwi Pear
Cherimoya Mango Plums
Cherries Nectarine

SWEET FRUIT

Bananas
Dates
Dried Fruit
Thompson & Muscat Grapes
Persimmon
Raisins

MELON

Cantaloupe Honey Dew
Casaba Persian
Crane Sharlyn
Crenshaw Watermelon

[Eat with no other fruit]

CARBOHYDRATES

Potatoes
Squash

[Not recommended: cooked beans, grains, grain products, e.g., bread, cereals and pasta]

OILY FRUIT

Avocado

[A superior source of essential fatty acids]

PROTEINS

Coconut Olives**
Nuts Seeds

[Not recommended: beef, butter, cheese, eggs, fish, fowl, milk, pork, soybeans, yogurt]

NON-STARCHY VEGETABLES

Asparagus Chard Green Beans** Spinach
Broccoli Collard Kale Sweet pepper**
Brussels Sprouts Cucumber** Kohl-rabi Turnips
Cabbage Eggplant** Lettuce Zucchini**
Celery Endive Parsley

MILDLY STARCHY VEGETABLES

Artichokes Beets Carrots Cauliflower Corn** Peas**

IRRITANTS – AVOID

Garlic Leeks Onions Radishes Scallions Shallots

GOOD

POOR

POOR

POOR

POOR

EXCELLENT

EXCELLENT

EXCELLENT

* Tomatoes only combine with non-starchy vegetables, seeds, nuts, olives, avocados, cucumbers and sweet peppers.

** Botanically classified as a fruit, but its bio-chemical composition places it in a non-fruit food combining category.

125

11

The Art and Science of Healthful Living

by T. C. Fry and David Klein

Natural Hygiene

Natural Hygiene is the art and science of living healthfully in accord with our natural biological heritage. Natural Hygiene embodies those principles which guide us to correct living practices. "Hygiene" is literally the science of health.

Our biological nature, i.e., the make-up (structure, function and living essence) of our bodies, determines our needs and how we should meet them. Health is our natural state of being. Disease processes (or illnesses) are perfectly natural responses enacted by the body for the purpose of detoxifying, rebalancing, adapting to harmful influences and healing. The condition of health (or wellness) is only achieved by living healthfully, i.e., satisfying our mental/emotional/physiological/spiritual needs.

Natural Hygiene, or Healthful Living, is about enhancing physical, emotional, mental and spiritual well-being through education and right living. It provides us with a simple, wholistic, living awareness system for regaining and maintaining superb human health and beauty. Hygiene is personally empowering and liberating. It teaches independence and rational action. It banishes fear and ignorance regarding human health and how to keep it. Ultimately it is about freedom.

Natural Hygiene always refers to nature as its mentor and teacher. When wholistic, comprehensive understanding is required, one must refer back to nature in her pristine majesty as the final authority. Because present-day life seems to be losing touch with those conditions which made life possible, Natural Hygiene brings us "back to the garden," so to speak. We should strive to meet life's requirements, and to smoothly balance them in all aspects so that we can easily lead a joyous and fulfilling existence.

Natural Hygiene concerns itself with those principles and truths applicable to human life so that we may wisely apply them to our lives. We are of the firm conviction that only by living healthfully can we realize the loftiest joys, peace of mind and blissful connection with all of creation which is our birthright.

Animals in nature are creatures of instinct. Following the guidance of instinct, they are correctly self-directed to meet their needs. They thrive optimally in accord with their environmental and genetic possibilities. Discovering and attuning to our natural instincts is part and parcel of Natural Hygiene. Our inborn guiding instincts always tend toward healthful and constructive living, when they are unclouded and given proper attention. It is ignorance of our instincts and the laws of life that creates our sickness and suffering.

In presenting the concept that health is normal and natural, Natural Hygienists emphatically refute the idea that disease is inevitable in our lives. We contend that disease will not occur unless there is sufficient cause. Health maintenance is an unceasing process in every organism. When the organism is overwhelmed by toxic substances beyond its ability to eliminate them in normal course, the body institutes emergency action to effect expulsion of the toxic burden. This crisis is called sickness or disease. Toxic materials accumulate in the body from two sources: 1) from unexpelled body wastes that are endogenously generated as a normal part of our metabolism, and 2) from exogenous materials ingested and partially or wholly retained due to inability to cope with the eliminative load.

We must eliminate the dead weight of false knowledge and ideas that we carry with us each moment. Using treatments, drugs, herbs, or anything else abnormal and unnatural to the body can interfere with healthful body functions but, under no circumstances can these agencies heal the body. Because these devitalizing agencies depress and suppress symptoms (or evidences) of body healing efforts, and because the body discontinues vital activities to contend with these agencies, which makes the symptoms disappear, the anti-vital effects of drugs and treatments are mistaken for healing effects. Nothing but the body can heal itself.

Disease is instituted by the body itself as an emergency measure to purify and repair itself. Modalities (treatments or therapies that involve drugs, herbs, manipulations, or other infringements upon the vital domain) cannot possibly assist the body. On the contrary, they interfere with vital body purification and reparative functions and normal body functions as well. Such interference poses additional problems for the body to cope with, thereby further lowering the body vitality. Body vitality may be lowered so much by the greater danger presented by the drugs or modalities that the original disease effort, which is actually an effort to purify the body, is discontinued in favor of devoting available energies to the more virulent enemy, the drugs within. That is why medical physicians are called allopaths. That is why there is so much "iatrogenic disease," meaning disease caused by treatments.

Allopath literally means opposite disease. In theory they strive to displace the original disease by creating a heteropathic or opposite disease. Actually all physicians succeed in doing is to create additional disease. The original problem remains while the body must redirect its energies partly or wholly to removing the more dangerous drugs, herbs, or so-called medicines. Thus symptoms of the original disease disappear (or are suppressed and masked) because the necessary energy and vitality to further conduct the disease is now lacking. Yet the body is in graver danger than before it was treated from both the uneliminated toxic accumulations and the added toxicity of drugs or other substances administered.

The best way to help the body in disease is to "intelligently do nothing" and simultaneously establish conditions of health-conditions that enable the body to devote all its vitality to the healing crisis. A thoroughgoing rest under tranquil circumstances constitutes a healing environment, for it permits full devotion of body energies to the emergency task.

The body is always acting intelligently and correctly. The body is always acting appropriately based on the conditions with which it must contend. We can interfere with its operations, but we cannot possibly help it other than by furnishing the normal needs of life consonant with existing body conditions.

The prime requisites of health

1. Love of Self
2. Healthy Self Image and Esteem
3. Passionate Love of All Life
4. Awareness
5. Intention
6. Inner Focus/Listening
7. Abidance by the Senses and Intuition
8. True Knowledge
9. Graceful, Grateful, Respectful, Generous Attitude
10. Organic, Vegan, Properly-combined Alive Raw Food Diet
11. Pure Water
12. Pure Air
13. Sunshine
14. Warm Climate
15. Fitness and Posture
16. Security and Peace of Mind
17. Rejuvenative Rest and Sleep
18. Heart-centered Self Nurturing
19. Sharing of Love
20. Relaxation
21. Humor
22. Creative Expression
23. Emotional Flow and Release
24. Rhythmic Movement
25. Musical Indulgence
26. Simple Lifestyle
27. Communing With Nature
28. Gardening
29. Service—Living Your Life's Purpose

30. Engagement in Self-improvement Challenges

By living hygienically, or healthfully, we are enabled to rejuvenate and reach our full health potential.

The Healthful Living Credo of Life

Attuning to our natural instincts and aligning with Nature is part and parcel of Healthful Living. We are of the firm conviction that only by living healthfully can we realize the loftiest joys and destiny which is are our birthright. Two centuries of unfailing results have proven Healthful Living, which is synonymous with Natural Hygiene, to be the true science of health and the greatest healthful living practice humanity has ever known.

Healthful Living holds that life should be meaningful and filled with beauty, love, kindness, goodness and happiness.

Healthful Living holds that we are naturally good, righteous, loving, sharing and virtuous, and that our exalted character will manifest under ideal life conditions.

Healthful Living holds that superlative well-being is normal to our existence and is necessary to the achievement of our highest potential.

Healthful Living holds that supreme human excellence can be realized only in those who embrace those precepts and practices which are productive of superb well-being.

Healthful Living, which encompasses all that bears upon human well-being, and which bases itself soundly upon the human biological and spiritual heritage, constitutes the way to realize the highest possible order of human existence.

Healthful Living is in harmony with nature, in accord with the principles of vital organic existence, correct in science, sound in philosophy, ethics, environment, economics, and animal rights, agreement with common sense, successful in practice and a blessing to human-kind.

Healthful Living recognizes that the human body is self-constructing, having developed from a fertilized ovum, that it is self-preserving, that it is self-defending and, through the mighty power and intelligence that constructed it, totally self-cleansing and self-repairing.

Healthful Living recognizes that the body maintains itself in perfect health, completely free of disease, if its needs are correctly met.

Healthful Living recognizes that humans are biologically and anatomically frugivores and are constitutionally, anatomically and aesthetically adapted to a diet of primarily fruits and, secondarily, nuts, seeds and vegetables. Ideally, they must be eaten in the fresh, raw, natural state in combinations that are compatible in digestive chemistry.

Healthful Living recognizes that diseases are caused by the body in response to improper life practices, especially dietary indiscretions. Illness proceeds from reduced nerve energy and consequent toxicosis from internally generated wastes, from ingested substances bearing or begetting toxicity, or from a combination of both. Insufficient nerve energy arises from dissipation, stress, overindulgence, excess or deficiency of the normal essentials of life, or not normal to it. Accordingly, recovery from sickness can be achieved only by removing the causes and establishing conditions favorable to recovery.

Healthful Living recognizes that a thoroughgoing rest, which includes fasting (physical, emotional, sensory, and physiologic rest), is the most favorable condition under which an ailing body can purify and restore itself.

Healthful Living, which teaches that exalted well-being can be attained and maintained only through biologically correct living practices, is not in any sense a healing art or a curing cult. It regards as mistaken and productive of much grief the idea that disease can be prevented or overcome by agencies abnormal to our natural being. Consequently, Healthful Living emphatically rejects drugs, medications, vaccinations and treatments because they undermine health by suppressing, disrupting or destroying vital body processes, functions, cells and tissues.

Therefore, Healthful Living regards body and mind as the inviolable sanctuary of an individual's being. Healthful Living holds that everyone has an unalienable right to have a pure and uncontaminated body, to be free of abnormal compulsions and restraints, and to be free to meet his or her needs as a responsible member of society.

Today, Healthful Living International leads the world in teaching Natural Hygiene and creating connective community for healthful living enthusiasts. Visit www.healthfullivingintl.org for information.

12
Tools For Success
Along The Raw Food Path
by David Klein and Dr. T. C. Fry

Notice to reader: In this chapter, all writings are by David Klein, except where noted otherwise.

Raw Food Lifestyle Success Tips

Education - Read books by Dr. Herbert Shelton and the other authors from our book list. If you are really ambitious, enroll in the Natural Hygiene Course. Learn the basics of our physiology, namely detoxification processes, healing requirements, raw food nutrition and digestion. Understand that it's a continuously unfolding process. Hire a diet coach if you need help. See Appendix C for a list of health education consultants.

Set goals - Set goals and write them down. Go back to the list and revise it as needed each night before you go to sleep. Visualize, affirm, take action, give yourself validation and reinforcement, and you will attain your goals.

Psychology - Feed your mind positive healthful thoughts. There are over 20 lifestyle factors, aside from nutrition, which need to be optimized in order to create vibrant health. Eat mindfully and eat to live; don't live to eat. Design your lifestyle to have a good, varied "diet" of activities that don't involve food intake.

Contemplation and meditation - The best if not the only way to access the answers from within—what, when and how to eat, as well as any other aspects of living—is to sit in silence. Tune in to your body's signals and its needs will be revealed.

Practice body awareness to overcome emotional overeating - Emotional body awareness helps us delve into reasons for overeating, which are typically a quest to fill an "emptiness" within or a resistance to feeling certain emotions. The Somatic Inquiry (presented later in this section) can help you accept certain emotions and learn how to locate and tune in to the love that is always present, waiting to "nourish" your emotional body.

Exercise - Exercise makes the whole dietary transition go better and better. Exercise improves will-power, digestion, and elimination. Exercise vigorously at least twice daily to create true hunger.

Mineralize - If you are not in peak vibrant health, a mineral deficiency could be a key part of the problem. Minerals act as co-factors for our enzymes, powering them for maximum efficiency. Food sources rich in minerals are fresh vegetable juices (e.g., carrot, celery, kale), rinsed sea vegetables (e.g., dulse), and tomatoes.

Peer support - Associate with other raw fooders via raw food pot lucks (try hosting your own), outings, phone and e-mail. Avoid non-supportive relationships.

BYO - Bring your own healthful food and drinks with you when you go to work, travel, visit friends, etc., so that you are always able to eat the way you want to eat.

Transition - Substitute cooked fat with raw fat. Avocados, nuts and seeds (raw or soaked overnight) are healthy, satisfying sources of fat. Try making nut and seed milks and cheeses.

Substitute salt with rinsed algaes, celery, and fresh or dried tomatoes.

Substitute cooked starch with raw corn, zucchini, summer squash and Jerusalem artichokes (sunchokes).

Always eat a bigger portion of raw with cooked food.

Have no more than one heavy meal per day if your energy is sub-par - If you have nuts or seeds, avoid avocado and starchy foods that day. If you have avocado, avoid nuts and seeds that day. If you have cooked starchy food, avoid nuts and seeds that day. Avocado combined with starchy foods is a fair combination but works for most people. Avoid nuts, seeds and avacados altogether if you are not feeling well.

Follow food combining rules - Eat sweet fruits only on an empty stomach. Don't eat them with or right after other foods, with this exception: sweet fruit combine well with greens, celery and cucumbers. Avoid eating fats/high protein foods (nuts and seeds) with starchy foods. Eat plenty of greens and/or cucumbers with heavy foods (fats, proteins and cooked foods).

Be passionate - It is the intention behind your thoughts and expression that seeds the success you desire. It is the emotional force that you attach to your thoughts and your expression that catalyzes your transition and rejuvenation process. Choose to become vibrantly healthy and be passionate about life! Interact with other passionate, health-minded people, learn from them and share your passion and joy with them.

Relax, be patient and accept what is - Nothing can be or needs to be any different than it is right now—this moment is perfect and you have done and are doing the best you can. Praise yourself for being where you are, having the courage and wisdom to be on the raw food path, and don't get down on yourself for any reason. If you stumble, get up, don't give up. Rome was not built in a day; be patient, focus on the good things in your life, and in due time the fruits of life will be yours!

* * *

Five Keys to Eating Sweet Fruit Meals

1. Exercise beforehand. Eating fruit (or any food) when we have no cellular need for the sugar and other nutrients can lead to metabolic problems. We need to create the need for nutrients (true hunger) by exercising.

2. Clean out with water beforehand (10 minutes or more before eating). A clean alimentary canal will promote optimal digestion; a soiled alimentary canal leads to fermentation of fruit sugars, mucus production, indigestion, and food drunkenness or fatigue.

3. Eat sweet fruits alone (mono or combo) or combine them

only with greens, celery and/or cucumbers (except melons—eat them alone). Sweet fruits digest and need to assimilate quickly. Sweet fruits (except melons) digest well with only the "neutral" green foods (i.e., food which are low in protein or starch and therefore do not require a long time for digestion in the stomach).

4. Wait six hours or more after eating nuts, seeds or starchy vegetables, or cooked food. Those heavy foods require hours of digestion in the stomach. Wait until the stomach and intestines have digested and passed those foods through before eating sweet fruits.

5. Eat sweet fruits with greens, celery and/or cucumbers to mitigate overeating on sweet fruits (if you have such a problem). Rather than filling up on the sweet fruits, eat a small portion of them, then some of the green foods—alternate handfuls or eat together as desired.

* * *

How To Overcome Any Gastric Distress When Beginning Your Natural Diet

When we start eating a lot more raw fruit and vegetables, existing stagnant putrid and fermentive, gaseous food matter is flushed out of the bowel due to the energizing effect of the raw sugars and the high fiber and water content. Also, when raw fruit sugars contact existing bacteria-laden morbid matter from cooked starches and meat and dairy products, the fruit sugars will ferment and gas will evolve. This will pass when the bowels are clean. If we do not follow food combining guidelines, fermentation and putrefaction will continue. Digestive difficulties during the initial transition/clean-out phase will be alleviated by eating very simple, properly combined foods. If that does not work, eating mono meals will help in every case. Raw salads with grated vegetables will help sweep out the bowels and eventually fruit sugar and protein foods will digest cleanly. Pure water, fruit juices and smoothies help us clean out as well. When the bowels are clean and the detoxification action calms down, digestion will be a quiet and thorough process as long as healthful eating principles are maintained. Remember: simple eating is always best

* * *

Twelve Reasons Why We Overeat and How to Overcome

1. We are malnourished—we eat nutrient-poor foods and are craving nutrients.

Tune in to your body's true needs and consume delicious mineral-rich, organically-grown fresh fruits and vegetables and, if you like, their juices.

2. We harbor the false idea that we will not obtain enough nutrients by having small meals of raw fruits and/or vegetables.

Understand that raw food nutrition is infinitely superior to your old diet of cooked foods—there is far more nutritional, health-promoting value in one apple than in a seven course meal of cooked food.

3. We are tired and are trying to stimulate our energy.

Understand that when we are tired, our primary need is for rest, not food, and food cannot digest well when we are tired. Eating when we are tired will only lead to enervation, toxemia and a worsening of fatigue.

4. We are not mindful or present while we eat.

Eat slowly and practice being aware/mindful/conscious and present in your body while you eat.

5. We do not want to feel a particular emotion.

Choose to accept, feel and be with the emotion. Allow it to dissipate, or expand, to flow through your body and beyond. Explore the "Somatic (or Emotional) Inquiry" (see below).

6. We want to feel the nurturing "mother love" that is lacking in our lives.

Choose to cease covering up your emotions and to release emotional contractions and you will begin to feel nurtured by the love that is always present within yourself.

7. *We feel and believe we are hungry when we are not—we are actually eating to fill up an emptiness.*

Choose to explore, accept and be with the emptiness. Meditation and the "Somatic Inquiry" can help.

8. *We feel bored and we eat recreationally.*

Develop enjoyable, purposeful and healthful activities away from the food or kitchen.

9. *We feel socially obligated.*

Choose to act healthfully and be in your power—choose to take the best possible care of your self at all times.

10. *We feel too thin when we are in the detoxification stage.*

Accept and love yourself as you are, and understand that by living and eating correctly your detoxification and weightloss period will eventually shift into a rebuilding phase, in which you will add healthy weight with larger muscles and enjoy higher vitality.

11. *We are not physically fit and are at the mercy of our sympathetic emotions.*

Keep physically fit—strong spine and fit body translates into a strong nervous system, self-esteem, will-power, and keener physical awareness so that you can discern your true needs for nourishment.

12. *We believe we can "get away with it" one more time.*

Ask yourself: "How is this food going to make me feel in a few minutes, and in a few hours, and tomorrow?" Think about how you want to feel and make the healthful choice, knowing that as you do, you are raising your level of well-being.

* * *

Getting to the Core of Your Appetites
via the Somatic Inquiry

Know thy self.
- Socrates

While preparing to write this article I sat down under a tree one day and made a list of reasons why people, including myself, eat. I stopped after I had identified 50 reasons, and over 40 were emotional in nature! Humans mostly eat out of emotional habit, equating their "appetite" with a strong message from their body that says: "Food! Feed me now and don't stop until I feel better!" Some people eat to satisfy this "appetite" believing they are filling a true need for nutrition, while others do so knowing that this is not the case.

You may believe you need to work on "controlling your appetite." When we recognize that we have an emotional eating problem, working on "controlling our appetite" rarely if ever works. The reason is we neither understand the nature of the "appetite" nor how to approach it. I do not believe that our "appetite" is something to control, but rather something to *understand.* Let's explore this and see how getting to the core of our reasons for eating can help us.

Understanding "appetites"

"Appetites" can be considered to be desires which arise from thoughts, memories and bodily needs. The needs can be physiological (nutrients/food/water/sunshine/exercise/rest/sleep), or emotional (comfort/security/love). Emotional eating can and sometimes does help us cope. However, food can never truly solve an emotional "appetite."

Essential and non-essential eating

There are only three essential reasons to eat: 1. to nourish our bodies when we experience true hunger; 2. to hydrate our bodies when we are thirsty; and 3. to fuel our bodies before and during rigorous work and exercise. Eating for any reason other than the three essentials is, to a greater or lesser degree, not healthful. How can we set ourselves free of unhealthful eating?

Body awareness

The key to healthful eating is mindful body awareness. This practice leads to self knowledge, which is the gateway to health, freedom and longevity. As conscious beings, we have the ability to develop our self-awareness on our pathway of self-mastery. With regard to eating, it is beneficial to observe our food cravings/appetites, food choices, the manner in which we eat, what our mind is doing while we eat, our emotions, and our body's sensations during and after we eat.

By practicing body awareness in a relaxed manner while we eat, we gain new insight about ourselves and our appetites. The magic of this is that as we come to know ourselves, we are constantly improving our ability to make healthful choices. Then, as our health blossoms, sickness becomes a thing of the past. We begin to feel great all the time, and we no longer stuff our stomach, intestines and colon, pollute our blood and brain, or waste our money on excess food. There is a tool for helping us become proficient at body awareness and getting to the core meanings of our "appetites." It is called...

The Somatic Inquiry

The Somatic Inquiry is a practice of sensing and observing the energetic presences and voids in and of the body, the inner terrain so to speak, and so discovering our true needs. In practicing the Somatic Inquiry you will naturally hone your ability to eat, live and care for yourself healthfully. By inquiring into your appetites you will gain a deeper understanding of their nature, so that you can discern what is and is not true hunger. After a while it becomes easy and natural to integrate the Somatic Inquiry into your life—just like sensing the outside air temperature and deciding how much clothing to wear.

Guidelines

Sit in quietude and develop an internal witness who silently and non-judgmentally observes everything about your self: your thoughts, emotions, sensations, circumstances, etc. In a relaxed manner, keep on observing and practicing being present in the body, every moment.

One or more times each day, while sitting in quietude, have the witness do a somatic inventory: From head to toe, or any direction, observe all of the qualities of the energies, sensations, feelings, emotions and voids you sense in your body. When you come to a strong or interesting presence, locate it in the body and delve or inquire into it via the Somatic Inquiry as follows: What is the temperature, shape, color, texture, density, space, movement of the energetic presence? Does it have a sound? Is there any message? If it is a void, can you delve into it? Stay with the energies or the void and delve deeper and deeper, without dwelling on or analyzing anything that comes up. A shift or resolution may occur as you sense-feel.

Keep practicing emotional-body awareness all day, even while talking to people at work or in any situation. Sense the energies in your body and accept whatever is there, observe how it wants to move and shift, and allow it all. Sometimes there will be a message in what we are feeling, and it'll be safe to express it to ourselves or others. When circumstances rule this out, we can always use our breath, exhaling deeply, allowing the emotional energy to flow through us, releasing it to the universe. Breathing is a great tool!

Practice the Somatic Inquiry when you have food cravings/appetites. Focus on the energies in and of the body. This helps us become comfortable with and accept the emotional body. This practice is about developing self knowledge—getting in touch with our true needs and appetites. Inquire into the nature of your "hunger appetite"—become aware of all of its sensations and feelings. Is it located in your stomach area? What do you feel? Tune in and observe the feelings and qualities—sense the energetic presence as a whole.

If you are having a "hunger appetite" in your belly, is your stomach region giving you a clear food signal? Maybe it is uncomfortable and just flexing. If you stay with it, the craving may shift and resolve to something else. If you drink a glass of water that flexing might go away and you will have learned that the flexing was not actually hunger. Maybe your stomach is empty and just wants love—eating is not the answer; food is not love, but caring for your emotional needs is loving. How can you distinguish a need for love from a need for food? Invite feelings of love in and see what happens.

If you sense something uncomfortable in the belly, or experience low energy and a "blue" mood, this can trigger a sense of weakness, low self-esteem, or neediness, leading to the habitual emotional response of eating sweets to boost your blood sugar, or fatty foods to fill up the sense of emptiness. Inquire into these feelings too. The healthful goal is to eat only to satisfy true hunger. What does that feel like? Explore and find out.

Do you have a feeling somewhere that is calling for a specific type of food? Locate it in your body and get to intimately know it. Does your body want something creamy, or tangy sweet, or semi-sweet, or salty, or crunchy, or chewy, or juicy, or a combination of those? Do you recognize the food it wants? If you do, and if it is available, observe the food—sniff it, peel it or break it open if necessary. Sniff in the aroma some more. If the food is totally appealing, deeply feel the pleasant sensations in your body, then slowly and consciously bite and chew it. As you eat, observe the sensations and how you feel as the food goes down. Relax into the eating and digestion process, stay tuned in and keep on observing how you feel. Continue to eat until you are satiated, following your body's signals that your stomach is sufficiently (not completely!) full. Your appetite may shift, or the taste may change. It's best not to eat past those "stop" signals. Put the remaining food in the refrigerator, compost it, or share it with a friend.

If you have difficulty with the process of getting in touch with your inner signals, this may indicate that you need to detox further, work with a coach, or just keep practicing on your own. Living on juices or water fasting helps clarify our windows of perception; emotional contractions/armoring and dense-body dullness will open up to heightened sensation and perception. Juicing and fasting also helps us overcome appetites for cooked food.

After you have finished eating, observe for several hours how you feel. Notice your energy, any pleasant and unpleasant feelings in your body, any indigestion. Do you feel happy, balanced, unbalanced, energized, sleepy, moody? Are you experiencing an appetite/craving? If yes, locate it in the body and inquire into it.

The use of self-knowledge

File away all of this information in your memory and refer to it the next time you sense an appetite or craving. As you continue sensing and observing your body and evaluating all of your experiences, you will optimize your progress on the healthful eating path!

I wish you expanding enjoyment in your explorations of the inner terrain. The Somatic Inquiry is the most empowering and transformational dietary tool I know of; it can be more enjoyable than any artificial entertainment or outer-world adventure because it is real, it is alive, and it takes you to new fascinating dimensions of the wonderful you!

* * *

Being Relaxed With the 100% Raw Food Diet Goal

How can a man's life keep its course
If he will not let it flow?
Those who flow as life flows know
They need no other force;
They feel no wear, they feel no tear,
They need no mending, no repair.
- Lao Tzu

Health is a journey, not a destination.
- Anonymous

The view is the path and the fruit.
- Taoist saying

Everyone is on a path which, despite our ideals and efforts, can only progress on its own terms and schedule. When we relax and allow our process to flow, life becomes easier. Conversely, pressuring ourselves about our eating goals always has a negative outcome. When we push ourselves to do anything before we are ready, emotional tension builds up and up until the plan backfires. If that happens, we can change our attitude and choose the easy path, knowing that we are always doing the best we can in any given moment...and this is not only good enough, it is superb!

No matter what your goal and no matter where you are on your path, you are always doing our best. Whether you are at 25%, 50%, 75% or 100% raw foods, you are still the same wonderfully special person, and you are fine just as you are. There is a certain mystique about being 100% raw, and the health benefits can be the greatest, however, in truth, you are always the same perfect spirit, regardless.

If your progress is slow or stuck, it's OK—that is where you need to be...it is impossible to be anywhere other than here and now! You'll achieve your desired results and become healthier and happier by accepting ourselves, appreciating your intentions and efforts, detaching from the judgmental inner and outer voices, and taking one comfortable step at a time when you are ready. However long it takes, weeks or decades, and whatever happens, it's all good, and it all has its important place in your process of self discovery.

When you do reach our lofty goals, whatever they are, you may feel that life is better than before, but you will learn this amazing truth: the goal is not a final destination, but merely a milestone on our journey of unfoldment.

In sum: by relaxing, being patient, and loving yourself as you are right now, you'll be able to enjoy the journey and the fruits along the path.

* * *

Personal Insight

If you're unclear
and don't know what you're craving,
what you need,
or which way to turn,
turn and tune within.

The answers bubble up from inside.

Sit in quietude,
relax, focus inward, listen, observe, contemplate, be present,
and go with what makes health sense.
Stay present in the healthful flow of life.

That is your practice.

* * *

How To Effectively Present
the Raw Food Diet Message

During the first few years of our raw food diet awakening, many of us become super enthusiastic about wanting to help everyone we know get and embrace the raw food message. And many of us rub people the wrong way with our zeal—I did in the beginning!

Fortified with raw food knowledge, we want to save the world, and to heal everyone who is sick and appears to be making them self sicker with SAD (Standard American Diet) eating. However, not everyone is open to being "saved" (maybe it's not yet their time). Despite our best intentions, most people need the freedom to figure out if the raw food diet approach is good for them. So it is usually best to "plant seeds," i.e., give information—show the acquaintance a copy of this book or *Living Nutrition Magazine* and perhaps invite them to a juice bar—IF he or she is open to listening and learning, and let go of the outcome, i.e., do not be attached to the result. Your "seeds" may need a while to germinate!

In order to help people with the raw food diet message, we need to have a few things in order to be effective. Here are a few tips for raw food message "gardeners":

Understand that the easiest way to get through to someone's head is through their heart: people want and *need* to be treated lovingly or caringly. When we try to help someone while we are anxious, haughty, irritated, or angry with them (or the world), the person will pick up on that, via your verbal, body language, or psychic communication, and they will feel as if they are being attacked. We need to be at ease and coming from our heart when we are educating and intending to help others.

Use the attitude that you are simply an educator (or "gardener") presenting wonderful information that has helped many many people. Do not force or preach the information—present it when the opportunity opens up and you sense no tension. To become an effective "raw food info presenter" it helps immensely to practice your message delivery by yourself or with a raw food friend.

Be congruent with your message—i.e., if you are ill and healing and do not yet appear to be a model of raw food health, be mindful that image sells, and if your message is bombastic, your image may repel. If you are healing, it is best to focus on *your own* health. When you become healthy and are glowing with vitality, then you will be better able to help others—your countenance will do the selling on its own!

Be aware of your own raw food attitude—avoid becoming a raw food fanatic. Remember: food is not life—raw food is simply one of many ingredients which together comprise the whole health recipe.

Be mindful when communicating with others, and remember that *angels fly high because they take themselves lightly.*

* * *

Are You Possessed of Courage?

by T. C. Fry

Perhaps you'll recall the refrain:

> Dare to be a Daniel;
> Dare to stand alone;
> Dare to have a purpose clear;
> Dare to make it known.

If within you resides even a modicum of courage, you'll rededicate yourself to being a modern Daniel. And you need not stand alone! Mutually we can create thousands, yea, millions of Daniels.

In you I'm sure is the spark of courage that will impel you to learn what is right for yourself and, with conviction and resolve, to do what you should do.

You will set as your goal personal excellence in all matters. You will strive to help your fellow beings open their eyes to the beacon of Natural Hygiene that they too may lead their lives in ways of righteousness.

As a modern Daniel you will not yield to injurious temptation and importunity. You will set an example for your fellow beings. You will become a living testimonial to the joys of living life on the plane our biological heritage decrees.

Dare you to be a Daniel? Do you dare to stand alone if need be? Do you have a purpose clear? Do you dare to make it known?

Become a Natural Hygienist in all that this implies. You'll grow in courage and dare to master yourself. And you'll win from your fellow beings the respect that that being a Daniel deserves.

* * *

Don't Quit

by T. C. Fry

When things go wrong, as they sometimes will,
When the road you're trudging seems all uphill,
When the funds are low and the debts are high,
And you want to smile, but you have to sigh,
When care is pressing you down a bit -
Rest if you must, but don't you quit.

Life is queer with its twists and turns,
As every one of us sometimes learns,
And many a person turns about
When they might have won had they stuck it out.
Don't give up though the pace seems slow -
You may succeed with another blow.

Often the struggler has given up
When he might have captured the victor's cup;
And he learned too late
when the night came down,
How close he was to the golden crown.

Success is failure turned inside out -
So stick to the fight when you're hardest hit,
It's when things seem worst that you mustn't quit.

13
Alive Raw Food Recipes
Compiled by David Klein

Recipes can be eye opening and most enjoyable, enriching social gatherings, while helping us transition to simpler eating. If you have trouble digesting complex recipes, follow the best food combining and eat simple meals. Some of the following recipes may not be for you—they are complex, some combining nuts or seeds with sweet fruit. These digest poorly for some people and fairly well for others, depending on the quantity eaten and personal digestive strength.

Recipes are not recommended for every meal, or for every day. Ultimately, the goal is to eat one to three perfectly combined, unprocessed foods per meal. Mono eating—eating one kind of food per meal until you are satiated—assures optimum digestion and internal cleanliness, helping us to create peak health. Unprocessed, fresh, ripe, organically grown, alive raw foods is the best way to go.

Mono Eating

A Gourmet Meal for a Nature Boy & Girl *by David Klein*
Get the nicest, most perfectly ripe fruit, such as cherimoya, mango, sapote, peach, nectarine. Sit under a tree. Sniff in the aroma of the most pleasing fruit. Meditate on the fragrance. Notice and pleasant sensations in your body. Peel the fruit and sniff in the aroma some more, allowing the pleasure sensations to spread. Slowly and consciously bite into the fruit, chew slowly, and be aware of the taste and energy sensations in your body. Stay present, spit the seeds far and wide, and enjoy the experience until you are satiated!

Drinks

Morning Glory *by Living Nutrition*
Ingredients
Several sweet oranges
1 pomegranate

Instructions
1. Slice the oranges and pomegranate in half.
2. Using a citrus press or other citrus juicer, juice the fruits, mix and enjoy!

Sunflower Seed Milk *by Living Nutrition*
Ingredients
1 cup hulled sunflower seeds, soaked for 12 hours then sprouted 24 to 36 hours, rinsed several times.
2 inch piece of banana, or 1 tbs. raw honey, or 2 dates
Handful of fresh basil
Purified water

Instructions
1. Add all ingredients to a blender, starting with 1 cup of water, adding more water after 1 min. to desired consistency.
2. Serve room temperature or chilled.

Hawaiian Dream Shake *by Living Nutrition*
Ingredients
Flesh from 1 pineapple
Flesh from approx. 1/2 of a mature coconut
Water from 1 coconut
Optional: ice

Instructions
1. Juice the pineapple.
2. Run the coconut flesh through a Champion juicer with the bank plate installed.

3. Blend all ingredients in a blender, adding ice if desired.

Grape-Celery Cooler *by Living Nutrition*

Juice your favorite sweet grapes. After the grapes, juice 1 or 2 celery stalks per glass. Stir and serve. Garnish with mint leaves if desired.

Ginger Ale *by Living Nutrition*

Juice white grapes, 1 or 2 stalks of celery celery and a 1/4-inch slice of fresh ginger root. Mix, chill and enjoy.

Almond Milk *by Living Nutrition*

Ingredients
3/4 cup of raw almonds, soaked overnight and rinsed
2 cups of cold purified water
1 date, skinned
Optional: raw carob powder

Instructions
1. Finely grind the almonds in a blender.
2. Add 1 cup of water and the date to the blender, blending for 1 min.
3. Slowly add the remaining water, blending for 1 more min. Optional: add carob powder to taste.
4. Strain the mixture and serve immediately.

Liquid Sunshine *by Living Nutrition*

Make fresh orange juice and wheatgrass juice. Add 1 oz. of wheatgrass juice per glass of orange juice and stir. This is the ultimate breakfast energizer!

Strawberry Shake *by Living Nutrition*

Ingredients
2 to 3 tbs. almonds, soaked overnight or 8 hours
1-1/2 cups purified water
2 med. bananas, frozen
6 large strawberries, frozen
Optional: 1 tbs. honey

Instructions
1. Place the almonds in a blender with just a little water and blend on low speed.
2. Add the remaining water and blend on high speed for 1-1/2 minutes.
3. Strain the almond milk if you like.
4. Add the remaining ingredients, blend and serve.

CocoVanilla Creme *by John Kohler*
Ingredients for 1-2 servings
2 young coconuts with soft flesh (typically found in Asian markets, they are shaved with flat bottoms and pointed tops)
1 whole vanilla bean

Instructions
1. Carefully open the coconuts and empty the liquid into a blender.
2. Scoop the soft white flesh out of the coconut, adding to the blender.
3. Add the whole vanilla bean to blender.
4. Mix until smooth, serve and enjoy!

Entrées

T. C.'s Super Salad *by T. C. Fry*
Ingredients (serves 4 to 6)
2 to 3 lbs. of tomatoes
4 med. or lg. avocados (or 1 lb. chopped or ground nuts or seeds)
4 stalks of celery
4 lg. red or yellow bell peppers
2 lbs. bok choy greens
1 grapefruit (optional)

Instructions
1. Dice the tomatoes, celery and bell peppers.
2. Quarter, peel and dice the avocados.

3. Cut up the bok choy.

4. Place all ingredients in a bowl and mix together.

5. Optional: squeeze the juice from the grapefruit over the salad and enjoy!

Holiday Loaf *by Living Nutrition*

Ingredients

1 batch of seed cheese (see recipe below)

1 ea. red and yellow bell peppers, chopped

1 cup sunflower seeds, ground

1 tbs. dulse flakes or kelp powder

1 green or red onion, chopped

1 handful of parsley

Instructions

1. Mix all ingredients together and form into a loaf, garnishing with parsley.

Seed Cheese *by Living Nutrition*

Ingredients

2 cups sunflower seeds

1 cup almonds

Fresh basil

1 tbs. lemon juice

1/4 sm. white onion, chopped

Optional: substitute fresh dill for fresh basil

Optional: parsley sprigs, paprika powder, orange slice

Instructions

1. Soak the seeds and almonds together for 12 hours.

2. Rinse well and allow to sprout for no more than 3 hours.

3. Add all ingredients to a food processor and process to a fine consistency.

Celery Slaw *by Dr. Douglas Graham*
Ingredients
1 large bunch of celery
2 red bell peppers
3 or 4 tomatoes
4 oz. of fresh walnuts

Instructions
1. Grate the celery and bell peppers and place in a bowl.
2. Blend the walnuts and tomatoes in a blender and use as a dressing.

Veggie Subs *by Betsy De Gress*
Ingredients
2 long red or yellow bell peppers, halved and seeded, lengthwise
1 avocado, mashed
3. 1 cup of sprouted seeds (broccoli, sunflower, buckwheat, alfalfa, etc.)
2 large carrots, shredded
1 cucumber, sliced thin lengthwise
2 dulse leaves, rinsed
2 leaves of Romaine or leaf lettuce

Instructions
1. Spread the mashed avocado inside one half of each bell pepper.
2. Partially fill the bell peppers with the carrots and seed sprouts.
3. Complete filling the peppers with layers of dulse, cucumber and lettuce.
4. Top the "subs" with the remaining pepper halves.

Mock Salmon Paté *by Katherine Dichter*
Ingredients
2 cups almonds, soaked overnight
1 cup celery, finely chopped (about 4 stalks)
1/2 cup green onions, chopped
1/4 cup water
2 med. or large carrots
3 tsp. lemon juice

Dulse flakes
Romaine lettuce
Parsley greens

Instructions

1. Run the almonds and carrots through a Champion juicer using the blank plate to make a smooth paté.
2. Mix all ingredients except lettuce together in a bowl, adding dulse flakes to taste.
3. Form into a rounded (or other shape) loaf and garnish with parsley greens.
4. Serve as a veggie spread or on lettuce leaves and wrap to make a "handwich."

Zucchini Linguini with Chunky Avocado Sauce *by Betsy De Gress*

Ingredients (1 - 2 servings)
1 large diameter zucchini
1 med. avocado
1 cup of 2 or 3 varieties of tomatoes
1 large red bell pepper
Optional: 3 - 5 fresh basil leaves, finely chopped
Optional: 1 tbs. fresh lemon juice
Optional: 1/4 clove of garlic, finely ground

Instructions

1. Cut the zucchini into 3-inch chunks and use a Veggie Spiralizer to make linguini. Place the linguini in a serving bowl.
2. Pit the avocado, scoop the flesh into a bowl, then mash with a fork until soft.
3. Slice the tomatoes into small chunks.
4. Core the bell pepper then finely dice.
5. Using a fork, mash the tomato, pepper, basil, lemon juice and garlic into the avocado.
6. Spoon the mixture over the linguini and serve with a salad.

Biogenic Burgers *by Bett Carstens*

Ingredients

2 cups fresh hulled sunflower seeds

1 sm. onion

1 lg. tomato, chopped

1/2 cup fresh herbs of choice

Dehydrated vegetable seasoning powder, e.g., onion/tomato/celery/parsley

Instructions

1. Soak the sunflower seeds for 8 to 10 hours in 6 cups of purified water.
2. Pour off the seed soak water, rinse thoroughly, and allow the seeds to sprout for 24 hours, rinsing once or twice.
3. Run the sunflower sprouts through a Champion juicer with the blank plate installed.
4. In a bowl, mix the ground seeds with the chopped vegetables and herbs.
5. Form the mixture into small patties and coat with vegetable seasoning.
6. Dehydrate at 115 oF for 5 to 7 hours, until the outside is crispy and the inside is still moist.
7. Serve warm, or cold. Will keep in a refrigerator for 2 to 3 days.

Stuffed Pepperinis *by Living Nutrition*

Ingredients

Red and yellow bell peppers

Zucchini

Tomatoes

Avocados

Celery

1/2 handful of whole leaf dulse

Optional: onion

Instructions

1. Core out the bell peppers.
2. Make zucchini linguini with a Veggie Spiralizer.

3. Soak and rinse the dulse, then squeeze the water out in your hand.

4. Finely chop the tomatoes, celery, dulse and onion.

5. Halve and pit the avocado, then scoop out the flesh into a mixing bowl.

6. Add the processed or chopped ingredients to the avocado and mix.

7. Stuff the bell peppers with the mixture and enjoy!

Avo-buttered Corn On The Cob *by Living Nutrition*
Ingredients
Corn on the cob, freshly shucked
Avocado, halved and pitted

Instructions
With the corn in one hand and the avocado in the other, smear the avocado over the corn kernels and enjoy! Best eaten barefooted!

Pepper-Corn Boats by Living Nutrition
Ingredients
2 or more fresh ears of corn
2 or more large red or yellow bell peppers
1 or more avocados, halved and pitted

Instructions
1. Using a knife, slice the corn kernels off of the cobs, collecting the kernels in a bowl.

2. Cut the bell peppers in half, length-wise, clean out the seeds, and remove the stems.

3. Remove the flesh form the avocado(s) and mix with the corn kernels.

4. Spoon the avocado-corn mixture onto the bell pepper halves and eat like a "handwich."

Carrocado Mash by Living Nutrition
Ingredients
6 to 8 lg. fresh carrots

1 lg. or 2 sm. ripe avocados
Optional: 1 to 2 cups of broccoli heads
Optional: 1 oz. whole dulse leaf
Optional: 1 large red or yellow bell pepper

Instructions
1. With the blank plate installed, run the carrots through a Champion juicer, collecting the juicy pulp in a bowl.
2. Remove the flesh from the avocado(s) and, using a fork, mash the avocado into the carrot pulp.
Optional: Run broccoli through a Champion juicer and add the juicy pulp into the carrot and mix.
Optional: Add the dulse and chopped bell pepper to the mixture.
Optional: Scoop out a bell pepper and stuff with the mixture.

Mango Salad by Betsy De Gress
Ingredients
4 ripe mangos, peeled and cubed
1/2 head Romaine or leaf lettuce
1/2 bunch cilantro, chopped
1 sweet red bell pepper, diced
2 leaves of rinsed dulse, chopped
1 lemon, juiced
Optional: 2 scallions, chopped

Instructions
1. Wash and tear the lettuce and place in a salad bowl.
2. To the salad bowl add 1/2 of the mango cubes, pepper, dulse and cilantro (scallions if desired)
3. Blend remaining mango with lemon juice in a blender and pour over salad as dressing.

Tasty Tacos by Marti Wheeler
Ingredients
Whole lettuce leaves
Avocados

Tomatoes
Cilantro
Sunflower sprouts (greens)
Salsa (see recipe in the following Dressings and Dips section)

Instructions
1. Place the lettuce leaves on a platter.
2. Quarter the avocado, slicing lengthwise, then slice each quarter twice more. Place the strips on a plate.
3. Cut the tomatoes into 1/2 inch strips and place them on a plate.
4. Remove the stems from the cilantro leaves and place in a bowl.
5. Place the sprouts in a bowl.
6. Place the salsa in a serving bowl.
7. Assemble the tacos by layering the ingredients on the lettuce leaves as desired, fold and enjoy!

Sprouts

Sweet Dried Teff Sprouts *by Living Nutrition*
Do you think that sprouts taste like straw? Try making your own dried teff sprouts—they are sweet and go with almost everything! Teff is a tiny brown grain. It is usually available in boxes at health food stores. If not in stock, ask the store to order them, specifying whole grain.

Instructions
1. Add 4 tbs. of whole grain teff to a clean sprouting jar with fine mesh cover.
2. Pour purified water to a depth of about 2 inches.
3. After about 4 hours, slowly drain off the water, and rinse twice more with purified water.
4. Allow to sprout for about 4 days indoors, using a fine mist spray to keep the sprouts moist.
5. On about the 4th or 5th day place the sprouting jar in the sun, or on your car dashboard for several hours, then they are ready to eat.

Germinated Sunflower and Pumpkin Seed Kernels *by Living Nutrition*

Using either hulled sunflower seeds or pumpkin seeds, soak a handful or more in a dish of water or a sprouting jar for 1 to 12 hours. Rinse and eat plain or add to salads. You can eat them any time after an hour of soaking. The longer they soak the easier they are to digest and better the chance for all seeds to germinate, but do not exceed 12 hours of soaking, as the seeds will drown due to lack of oxygen. After germination begins the seeds can be kept out in the kitchen for later eating or kept in a refrigerator where they will keep for up to 3 days. Always keep them moist by rinsing or using a spray bottle. When bitter, they are too mature to be eaten.

Flax Seed Porridge *by Living Nutrition*

Place several spoonfuls of whole flax seeds in a dish. Slowly add water to just cover the seeds. Return in 1/2 hour and add more water, repeating as necessary to just barely wet the upper seeds to achieve a firm consistency that is not too watery. The seeds release a clear, sticky, tasteless mucilage which cannot be washed away, making a nice gooey porridge. Avoid soaking for more than 12 hours to avoid oxygen starvation—eat immediately, or dehydrate into crackers.

Sunflower Greens *by Living Nutrition*

Items
1 lb. or more of sunflower seeds in the shell
1 cafeteria tray
Organic dirt
Newspaper sheets
Water

Instructions
1. Place dirt on tray and level it.
2. Densely add sunflower seeds over the dirt, lightly pressing them down.
3. Thoroughly water the seeds.
4. Cover with newspaper sheets

5. Repeat watering every day.

6. On the third day remove the newspaper and place the tray of sprouts in the sun, continuing the watering.

7. Allow the sprouts to grow to a height of approximately 3 inches. The green leaves are tastiest during their initial growth phase. During their next growth phase a third leave forms and the sprout becomes bitter—it's too late to eat them at this time.

Treats

Medjhool Hors d'oeuvres *by Living Nutrition*
Ingredients
Soft medjhool dates
Slicing cucumbers

Instructions
1. Pit the dates and slice in half.
2. Slice the cucumbers into thin discs. Optional: peel the skins first. If the skins are waxed, peeling is mandatory.
3. Place the dates halves on the cuke slices.
4. Serve on a party platter, with or without tooth picks.

Sesame Hors d'oeuvres *by Living Nutrition*
Ingredients
Raw sesame tahini
Slicing cucumbers

Instructions
1. Slice the cucumbers into thin discs. Optional: peel the skins first. If the skins are waxed, peeling is mandatory.
2. Spoon a portion of the tahini on the cuke slices. Optional: place a cuke slice on top of the tahini, making a mini sandwich.
3. Serve on a party platter.

Charoses *by Living Nutrition*
Ingredients
Approx. 5 small apples
1 cup of fresh walnuts or soaked almonds
1/2 cup of red or Concord grapes, juiced
Cinnamon or nutmeg powder

Instructions
1. Coarsely chop the apples.
2. Coarsely chop the nuts.
3. Mix the apples and nuts in a bowl, adding grape juice and spices to taste.

Banana-Date Treats *by Betsy De Gress*
Ingredients
Ripe bananas, frozen
Large medjhool dates

Instructions
1. Slice in half and pit the dates.
2. Arrange the date halves on a platter or individual serving plates
3. Run the frozen bananas through a Champion juicer using the blank plate, or process in a food processor.
4. Immediately spoon banana ice cream onto each date half and enjoy.
Optional: Blend the banana ice cream with cinnamon, nutmeg and/ or cloves or vanilla bean.

Gooey Mint Cookies *by Living Nutrition*
Ingredients
2 cups of dried black mission figs (soaked in water if they are not pliable)
1 cup of soaked almonds
Several fresh mint leaves, shredded

Instructions
1. Process or run all ingredients through a Champion juicer.
162

2. Mix all together.
3. Form the mixture into cookies or balls.

Halvah *by Living Nutrition*
Ingredients
1/2 cup sesame seeds
1/2 cup almonds
2 tbs. honey
Optional: 1 tsp. vanilla
Optional: 1 tbs. raw carob powder

Instructions
1. Grind the sesame seeds to a fine consistency.
2. Finely process the almonds, or run them through a Champion juicer with the blank plate installed.
3. Mix the processed seeds and nuts together in a bowl, dribbling in the honey until you get a sticky mass. Optional: add the vanilla if desired.
4. For a "chocolate" halvah, mix in raw carob powder. Do not mix well so as to allow it to become marbled.
5. Line an approx. 3 by 4 inch box with waxed paper and press in the mixture.
6. Refrigerate for approx. one hour, slice into cubes and enjoy!

Plum-Peach Sherbet *by Living Nutrition*
If you have an abundance of ripe plums and peaches and fruit sherbet loving kids (or adults!), run the fruit through your juicer and collect the juice in a plastic container. Seal the top and freeze overnight. Eat with a firm spoon the next time a cool treat is desired, especially on a hot day. Experiment with other combinations, e.g., berries, pears, nectarines, grapes, etc.

Choconilla Ice Cream *by Living Nutrition*
Ingredients
6 or more ripe bananas, frozen
1 cup or more dried black mission figs. (If they are not soft and pliable, soak them in purified water for 10 minutes.)

Instructions
1. Using a Champion juicer, chill the rotor blade and blank plate in the freezer, then install them.
2. Run the bananas then the figs through the juicer.

Date Balls *by Paul Nison*
Ingredients
1 cup almond butter
2 cups soft dates, pitted
1 - 2 oz. water
2 oz. raw sesame seeds

Instructions
1. Mix the almond butter and dates, adding water for desired consistency.
2. Roll into balls.
3. Roll the balls in a small bowl filled with the sesame seeds then serve.

Peach Parfait *by Living Nutrition*
Ingredients
6 frozen Babcock peaches, in 1 inch slices
2 frozen bananas, in 2 inch chunks
Fresh strawberries or blueberries

Instructions
1. Run the peaches and bananas through a Champion juicer with the bank plate installed, alternating chunks of peach and banana. Optional: add a few strawberries or blueberries as you process.
2. Serve in chilled fruit goblets or dishes, topped with sliced strawberries or blueberries.

Fig Bars *by Katherine Dichter*
Ingredients
 2 cups dried figs, unsoaked
1 cup dried coconut
1 tbs. honey

164

1 tsp. vanilla
1/2 cup almonds, soaked overnight or 8 hours

Instructions
1. Process the figs in a food processor.
2. In the processor, mix in the coconut, honey and vanilla.
3. Spoon the mixture onto a shallow 8 by 8-inch pan, then score into squares.
4. Place one almond on each square.
5. Refrigerate 1/2 hour before serving. Will keep 1 day in the refrigerator.

Banana Ice Cream Sandwiches *by Living Nutrition*
Ingredients
Almond butter, or substitute whole raw almonds
Soft medjhool dates, pitted
Frozen bananas

Instructions
1. Mix equal portions of almond butter, or ground almonds, with dates in a mixing bowl.
2. Spoon the almond-date mixture onto a flat pan, then shape it into a large, flat square approximately. 1/2-inch thick.
3. Score the almond-date sheet, making approximately 4 inch by 4 inch squares.
4. Make banana ice cream using a Champion juicer or food processor.
5. Spoon some banana ice cream on top of an almond-date square. Eat open faced, or place another almond-date square on top to make a sandwich and enjoy!

Sweet 'n Crunchy Zucchini Chips *by Living Nutrition*
Do you have too many zucchinis and wondering what to do with them all? Try making chips!

Instructions
1. Slice zucchini into 1/4-inch "chips."
2. Dry the chips in a food dehydrator.

3. Eat the chips plain, dip into avocado or guacamole, or add to cold raw soups or salads.

Dressings and Dips

Mono Dressings *by Living Nutrition*
If you don't like preparing food and want to keep it simple, chop up your choice of avocado and/or tomato and add to your salads. Or, squeeze a slice of lemon or grapefruit over your salad. This way you make dressing in your mouth as you chew!

Deep Green Salad Dressing *by Betsy De Gress*
Ingredients
1/2 cup tomato, cherry or heirloom
1/2 cup fresh parsley
1 stalk celery
1 sm. or med. red bell pepper
1/4 cup soft nuts (walnuts, pine nuts, pecans, or soaked almonds)
Choice of crushed bell pepper, organic herbs, garlic, etc. per desired taste

Instructions
1. In a blender, puree the tomato.
2. Add celery and pepper then blend till smooth.
3. Add nuts and parsley and blend till smooth.
4. Add the flavorings of choice.
5. Add more parsley or nuts as needed to thicken.
6. Mix well into a garden salad.

Wholey Guacamole! *by Living Nutrition*
Ingredients
2 ripe avocados
2 tbs. onion
1 clove of garlic, minced
1/2 red bell pepper, sliced
1 tomato, sliced into chunks
Niblets from 1 ear of fresh corn
1 tbs. lime or lemon juice

Instructions
1. Scoop the avocado flesh into a mixing bowl.
2. Process the onion, garlic, bell pepper, tomato and celery, or finely chop with a knife.
3. Mash the avocado with a fork, blending in the processed ingredients, corn niblets and lime or lemon juice.
3. Serve with veggie sticks or dehydrated corn chips.

Super Pecan Dressing or Dip *by Living Nutrition*
Ingredients
3 to 4 tomatillos (or juice from a sm. lime)
1 grapefruit, juiced
1/2 pt. of cherry tomatoes
4 to 5 stalks of celery, cut into pieces
6 oz. of shelled pecans

Instructions
1. Remove the skins of the tomatillos.
2. Add the skinned tomatillos (or lime juice) and tomatoes to a blender and blend till liquefied, then add some celery and continue to blend.
3. Stop the blender and taste the mixture. If too sweet or acid, add more celery to taste.
4. When the desired taste is achieved, slowly blend in the pecans.

Creamy Italian Dressing *by Phyllis Avery*
Ingredients
1/8 cup lemon juice
1/2 inch slice of leek, chopped
1 tomato, quartered
1 tsp. minced fresh oregano
1 red or yellow bell pepper, cored and quartered
1 sm. avocado

Instructions
1. Place all ingredients to a blender and blend until smooth.

Creamy Cucumber Dressing *by Phyllis Avery*
Ingredients
Juice from 1/2 pink grapefruit
1 med. cucumber, peeled and chopped
1/2 cup ground fresh walnuts

Instructions
1. Blend until smooth

Tomacado Dressing *by Living Nutrition*
Ingredients
2 avocados
1 lg. tomato, diced
1 green onion, minced
1 tsp. dehydrated herb flakes or powder
2 tsp. fresh lemon juice
2 to 4 celery stalks

Instructions
1. Juice the celery stalks.
2. Blend all ingredients in a bowl, adding celery juice to desired consistency.

Carrocado Dressing *by Living Nutrition*
Ingredients
4 to 6 carrots
1 avocado

Instructions
1. Juice the carrots.
2. Blend the carrot juice and avocado in a bowl.

Cucado Dressing *by Living Nutrition*
Ingredients
1 lg. cucumber
1/2 avocado
1 tsp. lemon juice

1 tsp. fresh dill

Instructions
1. Blend all ingredients in a blender and serve.

Zesty Salsa *by Living Nutrition*
Ingredients
Avocados
Tomatoes
Choice of cilantro, scallions, onions, dulse flakes

Instructions
1. Blend in a blender

Pistachio Salsa *by T. C. Fry*
Ingredients for Salsa
8 oz. of pistachios
2 lbs. of tomatoes, cherry tomatoes and/or others
4 tomatillos for a remarkable Mexican flavor
3 stalks of celery
2 red bell peppers
Ingredients for Platter Bed and Dippers
Lettuce leaves
4 to 6 stalks of celery
2 cucumbers

Instructions
1. Chop about 28 ounces of the tomatoes and add to a bowl.
2. Add about 4 ounces of the tomatoes, preferably cherry, to a blender.
3. Cut up and add the tomatillos to the blender.
4. Blend the tomatoes and tomatillos then add to the bowl with the cut tomatoes.
5. Dice 3 stalks of celery and add to the bowl.
6. Mix in the pistachios and stir well.
7. Cut the red bell peppers into 2-inch pieces.
8. Cut the remaining celery into 2 to 4-inch pieces.

9. Slice the cucumbers.

10. Spread the lettuce leaves over a plate or platter.

11. Serve the salsa over the lettuce leaves, using the bell pepper and celery pieces as dippers and enjoy!

Sunflower Seed Dressing/Spread *by Katherine Dichter*
Ingredients
1 cup raw sunflower seeds
1/2 to 1 lemon, juiced
1 sm. handful of fresh basil or dill
1-1/2 cups of purified water (use less for spread)

Instructions
1. Soak the sunflower seeds in purified water overnight, drain then rinse.
2. Grind the seeds in a blender, slowly adding the water for desired consistency, then basil or dill.

Seasonings

Lemon-Celery Seasoning *by Art Baker*
Forget salty, toxic, dead tamari, Bragg Liquid Aminos, namu shoyu, soy sauce and other bottled seasonings and try this instead: Dehydrate celery and lemon slices. As the celery dries out, it hardens and becomes thin floss. Cut the rind off of the dehydrated lemon and discard. Place the celery and lemon in a coffee grinder and pulverize into powder. This is very salty, with a slight celery flavor, making it a great addition to guacamole, salsa, raw soups, raw crackers, etc.

Dehydrated Tomato *by Living Nutrition*
Slice tomatoes, dehydrate them in the sun or in a dehydrator, then add to salads. To make a zesty paste, rehydrate them in a bowl of water, then blend with some fresh tomatoes and/or your choice of vegetables.

Appendix A

About the Authors

by David Klein

Dr. T. C. Fry

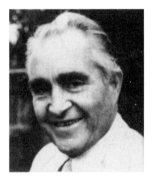

The Natural Hygiene movement lost its clearest voice, most brilliant writer and most prolific health counselor with the passing of T. C. Fry on September 9, 1996. T. C. Fry was 70. He left far too early, and his death was a shock to many whose lives he touched with his compassionate high-spirited ways.

There were many details regarding T. C. Fry's death, but in perspective the cause was overwork; he did not take the thorough rest he needed to heal the wear and tear of an active and, in later years, unbalanced lifestyle. T. C. Fry was probably more passionate than anyone on the health scene in getting the message out to health seekers about how to eat their natural diet and live healthfully.

It was in 1970 when T. C. Fry made his "great health discovery" in his reading Naturopathic Doctor Herbert Shelton's *Superior Nutrition,* wherein the principles of Natural Hygiene are revealed. He instantly adopted a hygienic lifestyle, overcame many long standing health problems and embarked on a path which lead him to become a giant on the health scene, teaching Natural Hygiene with devoted fervor.

T. C. Fry was a voracious researcher and scholar of the sciences of nutrition, physiology and healing. He put all his wealth of information into guiding thousands from illness to health, and his work saved many lives, including this writer's. He usually did it for little or no compensation, and what profits he did earn he usually put back into the printing and mailing out of more of his literature to health seekers.

A twelfth grade dropout, T. C. Fry was entirely self-taught, with Dr. Shelton's works as his foundation. "It's better to be ignorant than to have learned so much that isn't so," was his favorite retort to those conventionally miseducated nutritionists and medical doctors whose criticisms and challenges he loved to face head on. By way of his keen intellect and eloquent speaking and writing skills, he made many people see things in a different light, a more truthful light.

Many people were introduced to T. C. Fry via his *Healthful Living* magazine which flourished in the 1980's to the tune of 30,000 subscribers at its peak. Many folks agree that *Healthful Living* was the most inspirational health periodical we've ever seen. T. C. Fry's articles were full of life, explained health remarkably clearly, and literally taught us how to think for ourselves, inspiring us to take the initiative we needed to live healthfully. *Healthful Living* was the forerunner of T. C. Fry's last magazine, *The Wellness Messenger*, both of which inspired the creation of *Living Nutrition Magazine*.

Also among T. C. Fry's enterprises were a hygienic fasting center in Texas, and his 1988 book, *The Great Aids Hoax*. He believed that Aids is "the most fiendish and murderous scam in history." Indeed, T. C. Fry lived by Dr. Shelton's bromide, "Let the truth be told even if the heavens fall." T. C. Fry also wrote several dozen health booklets which he compiled in his "Basic Health Library," and he produced videos.

T. C. Fry's greatest contribution was the 108-lesson *Life Sci-*

ence/Natural Hygiene Course he masterminded in 1982 and offered through the Life Science Institute in Texas, for which he originally served as President. Many believe that the course stands as the most factual/informative/readily understandable/practical/beneficial course in the life sciences the modern world has ever seen, encompassing nutrition, health and healing. The course originally offered a Ph. D. which required a 6-month internship and a 15-day water fast (the greatest lessons in physiology/healing and the best preparation for fasting others are gained by fasting oneself). The Life Science Institute graduated 4000 students, including *Fit for Life* authors Marilyn and Harvey Diamond, and the world-renowned motivational teacher author, Anthony Robbins. The course is reportedly also being taught today at a medical school in France.

In 1983 when I was very ill with colitis and didn't think I would live much longer, it was my greatest fortune to have discovered a Doctor of Natural Hygiene, Laurence Galant, trained by T. C. Fry. Laurence introduced me to Natural Hygiene and T. C. Fry's course. One glorious night after studying the course I beheld a healing vision and the picture of my new health was revealed via T. C. Fry's teachings of the fruitarian pathway to self-mastery. The next day, in one fell swoop I changed my diet and lifestyle, and within six weeks I was symptom free! And free of medicines and doctors for good! During the next few years I worked diligently at re-building my depleted body, and when the times got tough I would call either Laurence or T. C. and find comfort in their affirming guidance. In 2001, T. C. Fry was given a posthumous honorary Doctor of Science degree by City University Los Angeles.

Over the years I have given silent thanks each day to this lion-hearted man for my new life, and we have stayed in touch. I will dearly miss our phone conversations, especially his big Texas-style "Well hello David!" greeting which always bowled me over with happiness. It was an honor to have shared his joy.

Many people miss T. C. Fry's joyous amiable ways, his high-spirited joke telling, his indomitable courage, and his unfaltering service when we needed health guidance. A while back, he gave me permission to reprint his writings. And so I will help keep alive his brilliant teachings to help many more people who are searching for the clear truth about how to heal and become healthy.

It was T. C. Fry's life work to reach all who were in need of his help, assisting them in healing and living a healthful lifestyle. He saw suffering and passionately worked to help people heal. He saw medical atrocities and boldly worked to right the wrong. The ultimate measure of his accomplishments are the living testimonials of those who, like myself, believe they owe their lives to him. In T. C. Fry's own words, he did it all "for a compassionate, caring, happy and healthy world."

* * *

David Klein

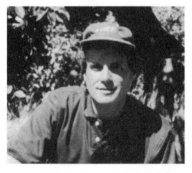

My journey into the health education field began in 1975, when at age 17 my robust health began to gradually decline. A heavy eater of meat and junk food, my physical and mental energies deteriorated over a period of six months, then I experienced incessant diarrhea. After a few weeks of medicine treatment, I showed little improvement, so a colon examination was done. The diagnosis was ulcerative colitis, and I spent my 18th birthday in a hospital, taking prednisone and azulfadine drug treatments. The symptoms subsided, temporarily, but the drugs further ruined my health and had a devastating effect on my mental abilities.

Within a few months, feeling sickly and very weak, I experienced a recurrence of the diarrhea and additional symptoms, including cramping, bleeding, and this lead to further physical deterioration. What ensued were eight tortuous years of colitis flare-ups and off-and-on drug therapy. At age 26, I was reduced to a weak, sickly shadow of my former self. I was having gastric explosions every time I ate, up to ten painful bowel movements a day with mucus and blood. My nervous system became shattered as I was toxic, debilitated by the medicines, and severely demineralized. Life became a dying hell, but I never gave in to the medical doctors' advice to accept my illness and just be patient until their impossible "miracle drug cure" came along; I desperately wanted my health back and doubted that the doctors knew what they were doing.

In 1984, I had the great fortune to find a Doctor of Natural Hygiene, Laurence Galant in Staten Island, who introduced me to the concepts of self-healing and eating a raw fruit-based diet. At first I thought the idea of eating mostly fruit while I was having non-stop diarrhea was crazy. Yet, I studied Natural Hygiene and slowly cleaned up my diet. I was attached to eating chicken and other favorite cooked foods, however, and was still having colitis flare-ups and relying on medicines.

In the fall of 1984 I had a colonoscopy exam which confirmed that I had advanced ulcerations throughout my sick colon. Surmising that I had been chronically sick and was not getting better, the gastroenterologist recommended that I either try his experimental drug which knocks out the immune system, or have my colon surgically removed. Upon hearing this, a heavy decisive thought entered my mind: I have had it with this medical madness—I'll be dead soon if I don't find the answer myself! My life was a gradual descent into hell and now I had to climb out now because I sensed it was almost too late.

Over the next few days I started thinking like never before about how to overcome my illness. I realized that I had to figure out what the MDs could not, and my thinking lead me to consider more closely the information on self-healing and switching to a raw food diet. The information seemed so incredible, but I saw that it was really working for Laurence, and I read many amazing healing testimonials.

Then one amazing night while studying T. C. Fry's *Life Science/Natural Hygiene Course*, I beheld a healing vision and it all made sense; the picture of my new health was revealed via the fruitarian pathway to self-mastery. I understood that humans are biologically fruit eaters, and that fruit was the best food for my sick colon. I was ecstatic knowing I had set myself free! The next day I threw away the medicines, divorced myself from all medical intervention for good, gave up all meat and dairy for ever and started a three-day juice cleanse. By the second day I was coming back to life. On the third day I was feeling better and better and my enthusiasm and joy drove my family and friends crazy! My gut was feeling soothed and I was rejuvenating. I set myself free of illness, doctors and medicines for good, and my bowels were working better and better!

I adopted a fruit based diet—that harmonized best with my mind/body/spirit. And with that my energies continuously increased as I detoxified and began rebuilding. Within about six weeks I felt that my colon was completely healed up. I was able to enjoy eating and life again, as my bowels were functioning better than ever. I began a new healthful lifestyle.

Over the next few years I diligently worked at rebuilding my depleted body, incorporating daily running and yoga, all the while studying the life sciences and all of the physical, mental, emotional and spiritual factors which determine our health. It took several years of total dedication to build robust health.

In 1993, after a year of study and training at the Institute for Educational Therapy in Cotati, California, I became certified as a Nutrition Educator and began providing nutrition and healing consultations. In 1996 I began publishing *Living Nutrition Magazine,* teaching health seekers how to eat our natural alive raw food diet, overcome illness the natural way, and live healthfully. I also direct Colitis & Crohn's Health Recovery Services and have authored the book *Self Healing Colitis & Crohn's*. I recently helped found Healthful Living International, the world's premier Natural Hygiene organization, led by professional health consultants and doctors. I also created the Fruitarian Worldwide Network. Today, at age 46, I enjoy excellent vibrant health and usually feel half my age.

Healing, I teach people, is easy if we understand and apply the principle that it is the body that does the healing—when we remove the unhealthful aspects of our diet and lifestyle and step out of the way, the body will do the healing work automatically and naturally.

Is living my 100% raw food fruitarian lifestyle hard? No! Living healthfully is the easiest and most joyful way to be! And I'm glad to help health seekers get there and feel that for themselves, and I wish you all the best in joyous health!

David Klein
Owner, Living Nutrition Publications
Publisher/Editor, Living Nutrition Magazine
Director, Colitis & Crohn's Health Recovery Services
Treasurer, Healthful Living International
Partner, Raw Passion Productions
Post Box 256, Sebastopol, CA 95473 USA
Phone: (707) 829-0362
www.livingnutrition.com
dave@livingnutrition.com
www.colitis-crohns.com
dave@colitis-crohns.com
www.healthfullivingintl.org
www.fruitariannetwork.com
www.selfhealingempowerment.com
www.raw-passion.com
www.rawstock.us

Appendix B

Further Education
by T. C. Fry and David Klein

*Your fellow Earth citizens desperately need
this message—
will you help them receive it?*

Obviously, our fellow Americans desperately need this message of health as over half of them suffer a chronic problem! You can get this message of health to your family members, relatives, acquaintances, neighbors, fellow church members, fellow workers and associates by acquiring additional copies of this booklet for distribution! We urge you to help NOW to end America's suffering and its trillion-dollar plus annual "health-care" bills.

You may order extra copies of *Your Natural Diet: Alive Raw Foods* from Living Nutrition. Individual copies are $15.00 each.

We also publish *Living Nutrition,* the world's premier raw food lifestyle magazine—teaching the natural way to eat and be healthy in this modern stress-filled world. *Living Nutrition* is a voice of Healthful Living International, coming out two times per year, with a writing staff of the world's leading raw health educators and doctors. Please visit the *Living Nutrition* online sampler at www. livingnutrition.com. Sample copies are $6.00 plus $2 postage ($4 postage for foreign orders). Subscription rates are:
5 issues: $24 U.S. - $38 Canada - $50 All other countries
8 issues: $35 U.S. - $58 Canada - $75 All other countries
12 issues: $50 U.S. - $78 Canada - $110 All other countries
20 issues: $75 U.S . - $120 Canada - $175 All other countries

Publications available from Living Nutrition:

- A Doctor's Raw Food Cure (Dr. Abramowski) $4.00
- Awakening Our Self Healing Body (Baker) $10.00 (discounted price - covers blemished)
- Children of the Sun (Kennedy) $15.00
- Dictionary of Natural Foods (Dr. Esser) $10.00
- Fasting Can Save Your Life (Dr. Shelton) $12.00
- Feel Good Food (Miller & Knowler) $18.00
- Food Combining Made Easy (Dr. Shelton) $5.00
- Fresh Vegetable and Fruit Juices (Dr. Walker) $8.00
- Fruit the Food & Medicine For Man (Krok) $15.00
- Fruit: The Ultimate Diet (Durette) $13.00
- Golden Path to Rejuvenation (Krok) $8.00
- Grain Damage (Dr. Graham) $7.00
- High Energy Methods (Fry) $36
- Living Nutrition's Favorite Alive Raw Food Recipes (LN) $8.00
- *Living Nutrition Magazine* $24 per 4 issues (U.S), ($36 foreign), back issues $6.00 each
- Natural Hygiene—The Pristine Way of Life (Dr. Shelton) $16.00
- On Nutrition and Physical Performance (Dr. Graham) $15.00
- Perfect Body book (Gallo) $17.95
- Perfect Body tape (Gallo) $10.00
- Primal Mothering in a Modern World (Halfmoon) $15.00
- Raw Family (Boutenkos) $15.00
- Raw Food Pearamid + Food Combining Poster (Klein) $8.00
- Raw Kids (Solomae) $14.00
- Self Healing Colitis & Crohn's (Klein) $19.95
- Self Healing Power! (Fry, Shelton, Klein) $10.00
- Sunlight (Kime) $20.00
- Superior Nutrition (Shelton) $12.00
- The Children's Health Food Book (Seaborn) $15.00
- The Essene Gospel of Peace (Szekely) $2.00
- The Fruits Of Healing—A Story About A Natural Healing Of Ulcerative Colitis (Klein) $5.00
- The Garden of Eden Raw Recipes (Avery) $12.00

- The Great AIDS Hoax (Fry) $4.00
- The Great Fruitarian Debate! (Fry) $7.00
- The High Energy Diet Recipe Guide (Graham) $12.00
- The High Energy Diet Video (Dr. Graham) $22.00
- The Raw Life (Nison) $20.00
- The Salt Conspiracy (Bidwell) $6.00
- The Science and Fine Art of Food and Nutrition (Dr. Shelton) $15.00
- The Seven Essentials for Overcoming Illness & Creating Ever lasting Wellness (Klein) $5.00
- Yoga Gave Me Superior Health (Bernard) $15.00
- Your Natural Diet: Alive Raw Foods (Fry & Klein) $15.00

For descriptions and selected book reviews, please see the Living Nutrition Online Bookstore at www.livingnutrition.com/bookstore.html

Notice to buyer: Prices subject to change.

U.S. postage and handling: $4.00 for first 2 items, and $0.50 for each additional item.

Foreign postage and handling: $10.00 for first 3 items, and $1.00 for each additional item.

Please make checks payable to: Living Nutrition, Post Box 256, Sebastopol, CA 95473 USA

Book and subscription order line: (707) 829-0362

Fax: (240) 414-5341

Online ordering: www.livingnutrition.com/bookstore.html

Customer service: 10:00 a.m. - 5:00 p.m. Pacific Standard Time

Major credit cards accepted

Appendix C

Healthful Resources

Appliances, Clothing and Fitness Equipment

Discount Juicers
John Kohler
Juicers, dehydrators, sprouters, water purifiers
(707) 581-1701
www.discountjuicers.com

Living Nutrition's Heath Shop
Stainless steel water distillers, Veggie Spiralizer, unfinished maple bowls, natural fiber shirts, glass drinking straws
(707) 829-0362
www.livingnutrition.com/goods.html

Planet Health
Ed Lieb
Rebounders
(800) 398-6237
www.sobehealthy.com

Rawganique
Natural fiber clothing
wwww.rawganique.com

UK Juicers
Nick Ledger
Juicers
North Yorks, England
www.ukjuicers.com

Waterwise
Water distillers, air filters
(800) 874-9028
www.waterwise.com

* * *

Ecological and Gardening Resources

**Earth Health Regeneration Orchard
and Gardening Services**
Don Weaver
Woodside, California
(650) 347-9693
earthdon@yahoo.com

Exotica Rare Fruit Tree Nursery
Vista, California
(760) 724-9093

Organic USA
Seattle, Washington
(800) 927-2527

Remineralize the Earth
reminearth@aol.com
www.remineralize-the-earth.org

Synergy Seeds
George Stevens
Somes Bar, California
www.synergyseeds.com

* * *

Health Education Consultants

Dr. Laurence Galant
Staten Island, New York
(718) 979-1889
newlifeinnovators@msn.com
www.newlifeinnovators.com

Roe Gallo, M.A., Ph.D.
San Francisco, California
roe@roegallo.com
www.roegallo.com

Douglas Graham, D.C.
Key Largo, Florida
(305) 743-8882
foodnsport@aol.com
www.foodnsport.com

Rozalind Gruben, A.H.S.I. , R.S.A.
Storrington, England
01903-746572
healthyunlimited@aol.com

Drs. Tosca and Gregory Haag
La Vernia, Texas
(830) 234-3488
drhaag@roylretreat.com
www.roylretreat.com

Healthful Living Educators
Healthful Living International
Sebastopol, California
(866) HLI-3HLI
www.heathfullivingintl.org

David Klein, B.S., N. Ed.
Sebastopol, California
(707) 829-0362
dave@livingnutrition.com
www.livingnutrition.com
www.colitis-crohns.com
www.selfhealingempowerment.com

Robert Sniadach, D.C.
rwsniadach@transformationinst.com
www.transformationinst.com

Thomas Stone, D.D.S.
Scotts Valley, California
(831) 458-6438

Timothy Trader, N.M.D.
drtim@attglobal.net

Vivian Virginia Vetrano, D.C, hM.D.
Barksdale, Texas
(830) 234-3499
vvvetrano@rionet.cc

* * *

Health Organizations

Colitis & Crohn's Health Recovery Services

David Klein
Sebastopol, California
(707) 829-0362
dave@colitis-crohns.com
www.colitis-crohns.com

Fresh Network

Karen Knowler
Ely, Cambs, England
44-0-870-800-7070
info@fresh-network.com
www.fresh-network.com

Fruitarian Worldwide Network

David Klein
www.fruitariannetwork.com

Healthful Living International

Dr. Douglas Graham, Rozalind Gruben, David Klein,
Dr. Robert Sniadach, Dr. Timothy Trader
Sebastopol, California
(866) HLI-3HLI
info@healthfullivingintl.com
www.healthfullivingintl.org
www.naturalhygiene.info

International Biogenic Society

Swallow
Nelson, B.C., Canada
(250) 357-9265

Self Healing Empowement

David Klein

Sebastopol, California

(707) 829-0362

www.selfhealingempowerment.com

Transformation Institute

Dr. Robert Sniadach

rwsniadach@transformationinst.com

www.transformationinst.com

* * *

Health Education Periodicals

Boletin Crudo

Balta Lorenzo

"Cortijo Crudo," Costa Tropical, Lista de Correos, 18690 Almunecar, Granada, Spain

Fruit Gardener

2609 Samarkand Dr., Santa Barbara, California 93105

(805) 682-2533

www.crfg.org

Get Fresh!

Karen Knowler

P.O. Box 71, Ely, Cambs, CB7 4GU England

44-0-870-800-7070

info@fresh-network.com

www.fresh-network.com

Hygienic Community Network News

Helen Jean Story

P.O. Box 1204, Santa Cruz, CA 95061

Living Nutrition Magazine
David Klein
P.O. Box 256, Sebastopol, California, 95473
(707) 829-0362
info@livingnutrition.com
www.livingnutrition.com

Vibrancy
Dr. Gina Shaw
ginashw@aol.com
www.vibrancy.homestead.com/pageone.html

* * *

Health Education and Professional Training Courses

High Energy Methods
T. C. Fry
Living Nutrition Bookstore
(707) 829-0362
www.livingnutrition.com/bookstore.html

Living Light Culinary Arts Institute
Cherie Soria
www.rawfoodchef.com

Natural Hygiene Home Study Courses
School of Natural Hygiene
Dr. Robert Sniadach
rwsniadach@transformationinst.com
www.transformationinst.com

Raw Nutritional Science Courses
Dr. Douglas Graham and Professor Rozalind Gruben
foodnsport@aol.com
www.foodnsport.com

* * *

Health Education Seminars and Festivals

Health and Fitness Sports Camps
Dr. Douglas Graham and Professor Rozalind Gruben
foodnsport@aol.com
healthyunlimited@aol.com
www.foodnsport.com

Portland Festival of Raw and Living Foods
Victoria Jayne
Portland, Oregon
www.rawfoods.com/festival

Raw Passion Seminars and Rawstock Festivals - Raw Passion Productions
David Klein and Dr. Douglas Graham
Sebastopol, California
(707) 829-0362
event@raw-passion.com
www.raw-passion.com
www.rawstock.us

Raw World
Cherie Soria and Dan Ladermann
www.rawworld.org

* * *

Health Retreats

La Via
Jim Horan
Aguanga, California
(909) 767-1096

Regency Health Resort and Spa
Dr. Frank Sabatino
Hallandale, Florida
(954) 454-2220
www.regencyhealthspa.com

School of Natural Hygiene
Dr. Robert Sniadach
www.transformationinst.com
rwsniadach@transformationinst.com

The Rest of Your Life Health Retreat
Drs. Grogory and Tosca Haag
La Vernia, Texas
(830) 234-3488
drhaag@roylretreat.com
www.roylretreat.com

* * *

Raw Food and Water Sources

Glaser Farms
Miami, Florida
(305) 238-7747

Jaffe Brothers
Valley Center, California
(760) 749-1133
www.organicfruitsandnuts.com

Living Nutrition
Sebastopol, California
(707) 829-0262
www.livingnutrition.com

Maine Coast Sea Vegetables
Franklin, Maine
(207) 565-2907
www.seaveg.com

The Date People
Jaime and Anjou Jones
Niland, California
(760) 359-3211

* * *

Raw Food Restaurants

Arnold's Way
319 W. Main St., Lansdale, Pennsylvania
(215) 361-0116
www.arnoldsway.com

Caravan of Dreams
405 E. 6th St., New York City, New York
(212) 254-1613

Roxanne's
320 Magnolia Ave., Larkspur, California
(415) 924-5004
www.roxraw.com

* * *

Web Resources

- **California Rare Fruit Growers Association** www.crfg.org
- **Colitis & Crohn's Health Recovery Services** - David Klein
  www.colitis-crohns.com
- **Discount Juicers - John Kohler** www.discountjuicers.com
- **Essence of Health - Morris Krok** www.essenceofhealth.net
- **Portland Festival of Raw & Living Foods**
  www.rawfoods.com/festival
- **Fresh Network - Karen Knowler** www.fresh-network.com
- **Fruitarian Worldwide Network** www.fruitariannetwork.com
- **Garden of Health - Karen Fierro** www.gardenofhealth.com
- **Gypsy Boots, King of Health** www.gypsyboots.com
- **Health and Fitness Sports Camps - Dr. Douglas Graham**
  www.foodnsport.com
- **Healthful Living International** www.healthfullivingintl.org
- **Living & Raw Foods Community - John Kohler**
  www.living-foods.com
- **Living Light Culinary Arts Institute - Cherie Soria**
  www.rawfoodchef.com
- **Living Nutrition Magazine Online Sampler and Bookstore -
  David Klein** www.livingnutrition.com
- **New Life Innovators - Dr. Laurence Galant**
  www.thruthinhealth.com
- **Ocean Blue Publishing - James Sloman**
  www.mayyoubehappy.com
- **Optimal Breathing - Mike White** www.breathing.com
- **Perfect Body - Roe Gallo** www.roegallo.com
- **Raw Family - The Boutkenos** www.rawfamily.com
- **Raw Food Potlucks Across America** www.livingnutrition.com/
  potlucks.html
- **Raw Life - Paul Nison** www.therawlife.com
- **Raw Passion** www.raw-passion.com
- **Raw World** www.rawworld.org

- **Rawstock** www.rawstock.us
- **Remineralize the Earth** www.remineralize.org
- **Self Healing Empowerment - David Klein**
  www.selfhealingempowerment.com
- **Shirley's Wellness Cafe - Natural Pet Care** www.shirleys-wellness-cafe.com
- **Steven King, King of Guitar** www.kingofguitar.net
- **The Raw Gourmet - Nomi Shannon** www.rawgourmet.com
- **Transformation Institute, School of Natural Hygiene, Natural Hygiene Courses - Dr. Robert Sniadach**
  www.transformationinst.com
- **True Health - Dr. Gina Shaw** www.vibrancy.homestead.com/pageone.html
- **U.K. Juicers - Nick Ledger** www.ukjuicers.com
- **Vegetarian USA - Peter Firk** www.vegetarianusa.com

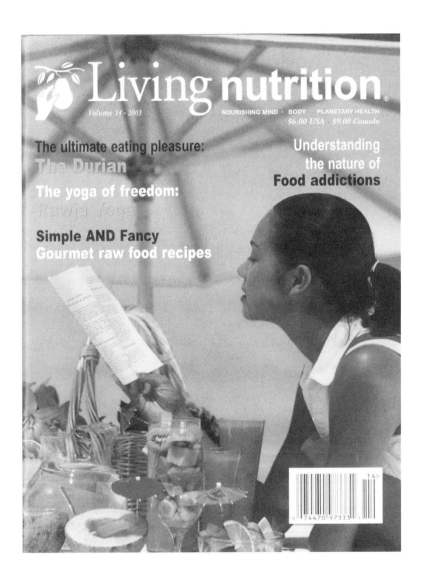

Living nutrition.

Volume 14 - 2003

NOURISHING MIND · BODY · PLANETARY HEALTH

$6.00 USA $9.00 Canada

The ultimate eating pleasure:
The Durian

The yoga of freedom:
Rawja Yoga

Simple AND Fancy
Gourmet raw food recipes

Understanding
the nature of
Food addictions

*Support your healthful lifestyle
with the raw food lifestyle magazine*

Living Nutrition®

The world's most progressive health magazine teaches how to eat our natural diet of fresh fruits, vegetables, nuts and seeds and be healthy in the modern world. *Living Nutrition* delivers a cornucopia of healthful raw food lifestyle inspiration, support and factual information with articles and interviews by and with many of the world's premier raw health education leaders.

Nutrition Education * Healthful Eating Guidelines * Raw Food Recipes * Natural Hygiene, Fasting and Self-healing Education * Healing Testimonials * Interviews * Physical and Mental Fitness * Yoga and Breathing * Meditation * Natural Parenting Education * Organic Gardening & Orcharding * Ecological Health * Food Safety News * Humor * Poetry * Event News * Crossword Puzzle
Published by David Klein every 6 months.

Samples of back issue copies:
$6.00 each plus $2.00 s&h in the US,
or $4.00 s&h for other countries

Subscription rates (shipping is included):

In the U.S.
5 issues: $24
8 issues: $35
12 issues: $50
20 issues: $75

Canada
5 issues: $38
8 issues: $58
12 issues: $78
20 issues: $120

All other countries
5 issues: $50
8 issues: $75
12 issues: $110
20 issues: $175

Orders
(707) 829-0362
customer@livingnutrition.com
or please visit our Web store at
www.livingnutrition.com

Living Nutrition
P.O. Box 256
Sebastopol, CA 95473 USA

"*Living Nutrition* is the crown jewel of the raw health movement. Not reading *Living Nutrition* is like not eating the heart of the watermelon. Stay on top of breaking raw food news, keep current with trends being created by raw leaders, get the best health education the world has to offer, and get totally inspired though *Living Nutrition Magazine*. It will uplift your life."
- Dr. Douglas Graham, President,
Healthful Living International

"The magazine is pure light magic!"
- Saskia Friedrich, Amagansett, New York

"*Living Nutrition* IS the most essential magazine around – way ahead of the rest. Indeed, it's the only magazine literally teeming with life!"
- Daniel Gish, England

Please visit our fabulous Web site:
www.livingnutrition.com

To request Living Nutrition's Cause of Health Catalog call:
(707) 829-0362

Live, learn and have fun with

Dr. Doug Graham
and Professor Rozalind Gruben

Health and Fitness Week
Raw Sports Camps

Fasting and Feasting
Every January in Costa Rica

Raw Nutritional Science Courses

"The best money I ever spent was on Health & Fitness Week.
It will change your life!"
Toni M. Cordas, Wilderness Ranger

"Sports camp allowed me to witness how effortless it is to
eat right and feel awesome."
David Leake, LaCanada, California

"I had the time of my life at Sports Camp! Find a way to make it happen
and meet me there next year–you won't regret it!"
Dan MacKinnon, USA

"Living with my health and fitness mentors at the Health and Fitness
Week was just what I needed to fine tune my regimen.
Healing has never been so much fun!"
Ryan Boley, Turlock, California

For event assistance and consultations, call or e-mail us:

(305) 852-0214

www.foodnsport.com
foodnsport@aol.com
healthyunlimited@aol.com

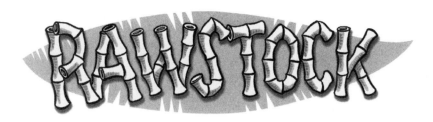

Pure health empowerment festivals celebrating
eco-regeneration, musical ecstasy & raw food delight

Next event:
August 28-30, 2004 in Sebastopol, California

**raw health, nutrition, ecology and organic permaculture
education * music * games * comedy * camping
fitness classes * yoga * tai chi * sport * canoeing *
community connection * joyous brother/sisterhood
* pure healthful fun**

Schedule and details:
www.rawstock.us
rawstock@raw-passion.com
(707) 829-0362

**If you'd like to join our Living Nutrition — Raw Passion —
Healthful Living International events e-mail list,
you can sign up by sending an e-mail to
58348-subscribe@zinester.com.**

Healthful Living International

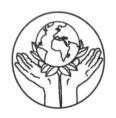

The world's premier
Natural Hygiene
organization

"for health, truth and liberty"

hwww.healthfullivingintl.org
www.naturalhygiene.info
(866) HLI-3HLI

DIET COUNSELING
&
SELF-HEALING
EMPOWERMENT
SESSIONS

with

David Klein, Healthful Living Educator

dave@livingnutrition.com

www.selfhealingempowerment.com

(707) 829-0362